PRAISE FOR JENI
CRACK THE CODE: UNLOCK YOUR FAT
BURNING & WEIGHT LOSS POTENTIAL

JNL has simply been nothing short of an inspiration to me. It is because of I am a Fat Loss Success Story and was featured on the cover of Oxygen Magazine and I haven't looked back. If I can do it you can do it!"

–Kimberly Castle *MS. TEXAS GLOBE 2013*

"Jennifer's candid and intriguing book "Crack the Code" equips fitness enthusiasts and beginners to "train smarter, not harder". It is important to collect legitimate resources for your health and fitness, and JNL has provided an ample library of information in her other books, especially "Crack the Code"! If you've hit a plateau or even need to review and be reminded of what is truly healthy and developmental to fitness growth and clean eating, this is the book for YOU!!" Jennifer Christianson-Blansfield, JNL Fusion Master Trainer & creator or "Survival of the Fittest, not the Thinnest"

–http://jdcblansfield.wix.com/blansfieldbombshell

"Crack the Code" by JNL is THE book that started it all! Its proven for fat burning and muscle toning, a complete program that will help you lose that darn stubborn fat, while toning sexy muscle, while not starving yourself. I suggest this to eveyrone looking to build the foundation of a powerful fat loss and health program."Unni Greene, author of "The Eat More to Lose More Diet"

–www.UnniGreene.com

JNL's "Crack the Code" is a must buy if you are starting out on your weight loss journey or are stagnant about losing stubborn fat. I love how it sculpted my physique and enhanced my sexy muscle tone. A must read for all!

–www.sandragonzalez.com

CRACK THE CODE:

UNLOCK YOUR FAT BURNING & WEIGHT LOSS POTENTIAL!

Blast Fat, Burn Calories, Rev Up Your
Metabolism, & Stoke Your Fat Burning
Furnace to Look & Feel Your Best

Jennifer Nicole Lee

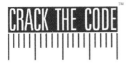

CRACK THE CODE: DISCLAIMER

MEDICAL DISCLAIMER The information is this work is in no way intended as medical advice or as a substitute for medical counseling. This publication contains the opinions and ideas of its author. It is intended to provide helpful and informative material on the subjects addressed in the publication. It is sold with the understanding that the author and publisher are not engaged in rendering medical, health, psychological, or any other kind of personal professional services in the book. If the reader requires personal medical, health, or other assistance or advice, a competent professional should be consulted. The author and publisher specifically disclaim all responsibility for any liability or loss, personal, or otherwise, that is incurred as a consequence, directly or indirectly of the use and application of the contents of this book. Before starting a weight loss plan, a new eating program, or beginning or modifying an exercise program, check with your physician to make sure that the changes are right for you.

Crack the Code ™: *Unlock Your Fat-Burning and Weight-Loss Potential* is intended to be used by healthy adults, ages eighteen and older, as a means toward incorporating healthy habits to achieve a fit lifestyle. This book is solely for informational and educational purposes and is not medical advice. Please consult a medical or health professional before you begin any new exercise, nutrition, or supplementation program or if you have questions about your health. Please keep in mind that results differ per individual, even among those who are using the same program.

ISBN: 0615808883
ISBN 13: 9780615808888

Jennifer Nicole Lee and Crack the Code™

After embarking on a personal journey to improve my health and increase my fitness level, I was named Ms. Bikini America 2005 and the first-ever Ms. Muscle & Fitness 2006. I appeared on "The Oprah Winfrey Show," "The Early Morning Show on CBS," "Inside Edition," and "ESPN." Then I became a personal trainer and top fitness model and was featured on numerous magazine covers and in articles. I enjoy using what I have learned to help other people achieve their own fitness goals.

Crack the Code™ is the first of many projects that will include merchandise, such as my JNL Fusion Workout Method, and JNL Fusion exercise DVDs, low-calorie cookbooks, fitness apparel, and fitness merchandise endorsements. I am able to engage my "fitness friends," as I like to call them, by writing from my expertise and life experiences. Like many women, I juggle being a mother, pursuing my career, and achieving my optimal physical potential.

I am a true weight-loss success story, shedding more than seventy pounds in under a year with my **Crack the Code™** principles. I took it to the next level. I proved myself when I was crowned Ms. Bikini America and then was named the first-ever Ms. Muscle & Fitness. Women want to look their best, even in their forties and fifties. I am here to tell you that the secret lies in strength training. This is the key element that helped me transform my physique to win my titles of Ms. Bikini America and Ms. Muscle & Fitness.

In *Crack the Code™*, I teach universal principles that will help both men and women achieve their fitness goals. I once weighed almost two hundred pounds. I can tell you that my principles have allowed me to stay successful at getting the weight off, looking and feeling great, and, most importantly, keeping it off for good, even through the ups and downs of life while raising two gorgeous boys.

In this book, you will learn how I melted off more than seventy pounds and transformed my physique after the birth of my second son. I reveal the number one secret to losing weight and keeping it off forever. You will learn my top rules for revving up your metabolism, losing fat pounds, gaining muscle, having more energy, stoking your fat-burning furnace, adding years to your life, and looking and feeling your best ever!

The **Crack the Code™** principles are solid and efficient methods for losing weight and feeling great. To quantum-leap your results and gain more clarity of the principles, go to www.fitnessmodelprogram.com, www.bikinimodelprogram.com, www.101thingsnottodo.com, www.shopjnl.com, and www.jnlmp3s.com.

Official Social Media Sites & Websites of Jennifer Nicole Lee

Instagram
#jnlworldwide

Celebrity Facebook Page
www.JenniferNicoleLeeFB.com

Official YouTube Channel
www.JNLYouTube.com

JNL Clothing
www.JNLClothing.com

The Fun Fit Foodie CookBook
Available at www.JNLBooks.com

The Fitness Model Diet Book
Available at www.ShopJNL.com

Mind Body & Soul Diet Program at www.MindBodyAndSoulDiet.com

Official Twitter Page www.Twitter.com/TheJNL

Get a Bikini Body Now at www.BikiniModelProgam.com

Book JNL to Speak at Your Next Event by Emailing TheJenniferNicoleLee@gmail.com

Want to Consult or get Top Coaching with JNL?
Then Apply at www.ClubJNL.com

Want Photos Like JNL's?
Then Apply at www.FitnessModelFactory.com

JNL's Wikipedia Page: http://en.wikipedia.org/wiki/Jennifer_Nicole_Lee

Mind Body and Soul Diet Online Coaching
www.MindBodyAndSoulDiet.com

THANK YOU'S

First and foremost I want to thank God for giving me the drive, passion, and resiliency to never give up and be strong enough to work towards achieving my goals for the greater good of all whom I may positively influence and touch. I also thank my amazing husband Edward for his undying support. And to my two sons Jaden and Dylan, I truly am the luckiest mom in the world to have you to enjoy every day!

To my entire staff and team members at JNL Worldwide, Inc, thank you for being so awesome to work with, always seeing my vision to all of my projects.

I want to give a special thanks to all of my JNL Fusion sisters around the world! JNL Nation is a very blessed, prosperous, and joyful global community of "believers" who will never give up! I believe in YOU!

I want to give special thanks to Coach "Wicked Willie" & Unni Greene, "The Diet Diva" for always believing in me!

Specials thanks to all of my JNL Fusion Master Trainers worldwide for being the best trainers! You are the best of the best! Second to none!

And a very special thanks to YOU! You reading this message right now! I want you to know that you have in your hands, and your eyes on something extremely powerful; this is only if you believe and you use this information found in this book!

I BELIEVE IN YOU!

Jennifer Nicole Lee

www.JenniferNicoleLee.com

DEDICATIONS

I started writing this book in 2003. Now its ten years later. Crack the Code was the first book that I have ever written, and first released as my first ever E-book. Now I'm celebrating the fact that its my 5th hard copy book. This goes to show you that I practice what I preach: to never give up, never give in, and always aim to win! I wrote this book out of my own personal frustrations of being fooled by and fitness industry. I spent countless hours in research and discovery to compile this complete lifestyle program. My "Crack the Code" book & program is one of the world's best fundamental systems which contains all the important elements to create a healthy, fun, fit and enjoyable level of wellness. This book is a powerful "weapon" on fighting and winning the war on fat! It contains all the basic, yet many times overlooked, "codes" of weight loss, that when put together "crack" open your fat loss potential. Also, it's been touted on by critics as a "must read" and a "must have" book in any fitness enthusiast's library of health books, because it contains the foundation of health and wellness.

I dedicate this book to all the believers, and to YOU reading this right now! I believe in YOU!

Jennifer Nicole Lee

www.JenniferNicoleLeeFB.com

TABLE OF CONTENTS

PART ONE: History, Preparation, and the Crack the Code™ Program

Chapter 1

Chapter 2

Chapter 3

Chapter 4

PART TWO: Stop Eating Accidentally! The Crack the Code™ Food Plan

Chapter 5

Chapter 6

PART THREE: Exercise Smarter, Not Harder: Get Maximum Results in Minimum Time

Chapter 7

Chapter 8

Appendix 1

Appendix 2

Appendix 3

Appendix 4

Appendix 5

About Jennifer Nicole Lee

WWW.SHOPJNL.COM

FOREWORD

by Unni Greene, The Diet Diva, C.M.T., C.S.N.S.

When Jennifer Nicole Lee asked me to write the Foreword to her "Crack the Code" book, I was deeply honored and very excited. JNL, as we know her by, is an enormously talented fitness and wellness guru whose accomplishments are almost mind boggling. She is the bestselling author of numerous books on fitness, wellness, cooking, exercise, diet and beauty. She is also a highly sought after motivational speaker, the creator of the JNL FUSION workout method, which has revolutionized the way people work out today, a life coach, the world's most highly publicized fitness cover model and, yes, there is more, the owner of several successful businesses such as The Fitness Model Factory, JNL FUSION GYM's and JNL Beauty and Wellness. She also earned the highly coveted spot as the official spokes model for the premium supplement brand, BodyFX. In addition to all this, JNL also gives her world famous JNL WORLD CONFERENCES, on an annual basis. These sold out events draw hundreds of fitness minded women from around the globe to come together to be empowered, learn from the best about fitness, nutrition, supplementation, self-development and marketing and branding from JNL and her Dream Team. Now, let me ask you, do you think JNL know about weight loss and fitness? You bet she does! With her demanding career and lifestyle, she still has to look her best, each and every day! And she does! JNL is always camera ready, as the paparazzi are constantly ready and waiting to catch a snap shot of this beauty! Not to mention her weekly bookings for photo shoots with the top fitness magazines. As a wife and devoted mother of two sons and a businesswoman, JNL has no time to spare. She has to do what works. In her "Crack the Code" book, she shares her hard-earned knowledge with us. And she has a lot of knowledge! You can trust that JNL knows what she is talking about. She herself has known the pain and frustration of being trapped in her own "fat suit". While she once weighed over 200 lbs., JNL shed 80 lbs. of fat to become the most highly sought after fitness model in the world. She did this through hard work, determination and by eating the right things at the right time. She learned what worked and what did not. In "Crack the Code"; she is sharing all her secrets on how to become lean, strong and sexy for life. All you need to know is in this book. As her long- time friend and business associate, I know what I am talking about. JNL coined me "The Diet Diva", due to my strong expertize in fitness and nutrition. I have four separate degrees in nutrition and I am a Certified Master Trainer and owner of my own private training facility. I counsel thousands of people around the globe and I am also the author of the bestselling book "Eat More To Lose More". I am blessed to be JNL's official nutrition coach, as well as the Official Nutrition and Exercise Coach to many well-known world champion athletes, celebrities and businesses, publications and TV shows, such as JanetTV. I myself am a mother of four and a fitness professional that also has to look my best every day. In "Crack the Code", you will find what you have always been looking for; simple, straightforward advice that works. It works for JNL and for thousands of women around the globe, and it will work for YOU! Happy reading!

www.UnniGreene.com

PART ONE:

History, Preparation, and the Crack the Code™ Program

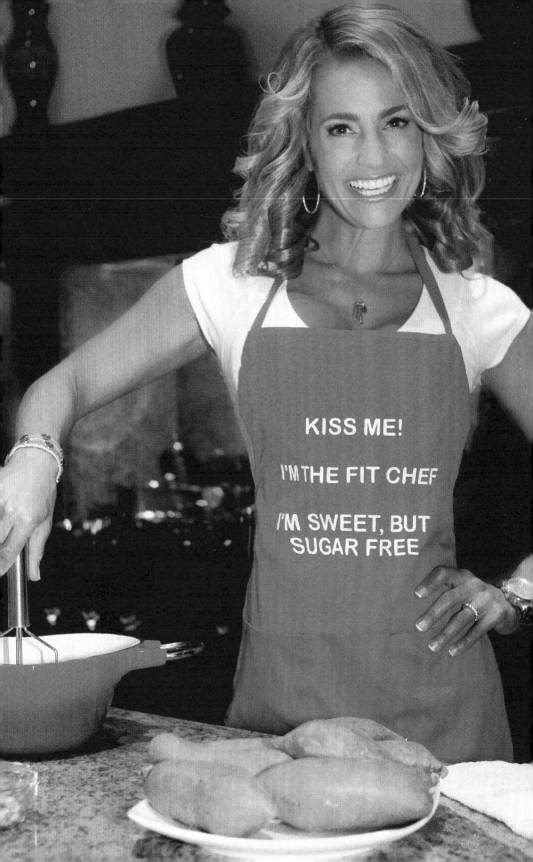

CHAPTER 1

Section 1: Yo-Yo Dieting through Life: How I Dealt with My Love/Hate Relationship with Food

"So what do you want to eat today?" This was my Italian family's favorite question. My mom and dad, being true Italians, bombarded my two older sisters, my younger brother, and me with food constantly. This food-focused question was the first thing they asked me when I woke up. Every morning, it was a serious topic of discussion over a fattening breakfast of fried eggs and sausage that Mom prepared with love. Sometimes, discussions over what the day's menu would entail ended in a heated debate; my sister wanted lasagna, while my brother wanted spaghetti, meatballs, and sausage. Eating was an all-day affair with no breaks. And no matter what I said, food was coming my way—and large portions of it!

Needless to say, my mom and dad showed their love through food. Well, what do you expect from an Italian family? The use of food as a medium for love was passed down from generation to generation, and it was the only thing they knew how to do.

Not only that, but I inherited the "fat gene." The correct medical term would be a slow metabolism. My slow metabolic rate further worsened because I was constantly surrounded by large portions and made poor food choices. Growing up, I gained and stored weight easily.

Do you ever feel that all you have to do to gain five pounds is just look at a piece of chocolate cake? Well, that was me!

We were always eating. My days consisted of one large, never-ending meal. And we ate for every occasion. Perhaps I should rephrase that by saying we did not "eat" but rather "pigged out" and "feasted." When we were happy, we would celebrate and eat. When we were sad, we would mourn and eat. When we were bored, we would eat. And when we were planning a special occasion, we would surround the event with food. It was always about food and what the next meal was going to be. After my parents separated, they graduated to "food wars." My mom would constantly ask me, "So whose lasagna is better, mine or your father's?" My dad would seem a little peeved if we went to his house on a full stomach from our mom's. He would ask, "So what did she feed you?" It seemed as though he was strategizing a plan to "one up" her with his next meal.

I was brainwashed, if you will, with the idea that food was truly the end all! And boy, did I yo-yo. The only fitness knowledge I had growing up was the starvation diet. I knew that I had to lose weight, but the only thing I did to achieve this was either not eat much or simply not eat at all. My body hoarded the fat pounds instead of losing them. And we have all been there—from Oprah Winfrey and her liquid diet to Princess Diana and her bouts of bulimia to many of today's celebrities going stick-skinny. Many of my clients have used "unhealthy" means to get "healthy." It is a crazy diet cycle that may have helped us temporarily lose weight but in the end only causes us to gain it all back—or more—after our diet ends!

Have you ever felt like a gerbil running on one of those stationary wheels, going nowhere fast? That's what the endless, unhealthy cycle of losing and gaining feels like. With my **Crack the Code™** program (also referred to as CTC) your outcome will be different! With CTC, you will transform your body into a fat-burning machine, unlocking your fat-burning and weight-loss potential because I will take you to the core of the problem: your metabolic rate.

In this miraculous book, you will learn so many tools that you will carry with you like a bag of tricks you can use at any time. I like to call it having ammunition with which to fight fat! I drastically changed all the associations I had been taught about food into positive tools I used to **Crack the Code™**. In doing so, I was able to transform my body into a fat-burning machine, unlocking my weight-loss potential primarily by stoking my metabolic rate.

Section 2: My "Aha" Moment: How I Finally "Cracked the Code" to My Weight Loss, and How You Can Do It, Too

I knew I was out of shape, but I could not imagine I looked that *bad*! It was an ordinary summer day but a day that changed my life forever. I will never forget it. It was mid-May, officially swimsuit season. A friend of mine was brave enough to take a picture of me in a fuchsia bikini. I didn't know it would be at the time, but this is now my famous "before" picture. After my brave and willing friend took the snapshot, I glanced at it. And then *it* happened. It was my "aha!" moment. I couldn't believe my eyes. Was that me? What had happened? Where had I gone?

I didn't recognize myself. I knew I was out of shape, but did I look that bad? Yes, I knew I was masking my weight by wearing bag, black clothes; lots of makeup; and big hair. But I stripped my daily costume away and placed myself in a bikini to get real. And boy, did I get real with myself. From that point on, I did all I could to lose the weight and get in shape. I placed that photograph in my bathroom so I could see it every day when I got ready in the morning. I saw it at night before I took my shower. There wasn't a day that I did not look at it and say to myself, "You can do better; this is not who you were meant to be. Realize your potential and work hard at achieving it. You can do it! If not now, then never!"

This get-real moment was fueled by other horror stories from moms at the park. One lady confided in me that ever since the birth of her baby, she had not been able to lose weight. I asked her how old her baby was, and she responded, "Oh, my son is five years old now." How could this be? Five years had passed with no weight loss.

This easily could have been me, but I devised my CTC program, complete with a sound food plan and exercise routine, to build lean muscle, melt off fat pounds, and add energy to my life, enabling me to look and feel my best! Now I am passing this wealth of information to you so that you may also get the energy, stamina, and endurance you need to get through your day.

My advice is to take a "before" picture of yourself and ask, "What can be better? What would I like to change?" You can improve the way you look with my CTC Principles, just as I did! I went from a miserable, overweight mom to being crowned Ms. Bikini America and Ms. Muscle & Fitness after the birth of my second son by using my CTC Principles. It all starts in your mind, and that is what we will address in the next chapter.

CHAPTER 2

Section 1: Free Your Mind, and Your Body Will Follow: Breaking the Emotional Ties to Food

Health starts in the mind and then flows to the body. In this chapter, I prep both the mind and body for the fantastic health advances that lie ahead. You must be 100 percent committed to making healthy progress if you are going to see and keep results! Although it may be hard to believe, sometimes we sabotage our own successes because we are not mentally ready and committed to sticking to our wonderful lifestyle improvements. You must create your results before they occur and prepare yourself for boundless energy and confidence.

To lose unwanted fat pounds, you must start with your mind! A close friend of mine sabotaged her weight-loss potential by saying to herself, "Why lose weight? My skin will only be flabby if I lose the amount of weight that I want." She had already set herself up for failure by predetermining that she was not going to lose weight.

A client of mine once claimed that she wanted to lose weight but was afraid of all the remarks from those close to her; she worried about how the change might affect her family. I told her that she would only be adding quality to her life, not taking away from it—and that these healthy new changes would actually be helping her family as well. In addition, this "fear" was rooted in the idea that she would never be able to lose weight. She worried about the added health risks of heart disease and diabetes, not to mention the added pressure on her joints from the additional weight.

These are examples of people riding the fence, not knowing what side to get down from. Make a decision to improve your life by being healthy. Your mind and body will thank you.

Section 2: Mental Preparation for the Whole Process: Getting Yourself Ready to Lose Weight

Start by asking yourself these questions: "Do I have a healthy mind, or a mind that will thwart my efforts? Am I my own best friend or my worst enemy?" If you chose the second option in those questions, we first need to clean your "mental" house! Here are my top seven strategies for giving yourself the right mental attitude that will allow you to start improving your life.

1. Have a crystal-clear vision of what you want to achieve. I have heard it so many times. My clients come to me and cry, "I'm sick and tired of being overweight!" or they complain, "I have no energy, and I'm tired all the time." This will not help you! We all know what we want to move away from. But what do we want to move toward?

I'm referring to the fact that we must realize where our main focus needs to be if we are to achieve weight-loss success from now on. We have all taken "before" picture of ourselves; now we need to have an "after" image of what we want. Envision what you want to achieve. See the new you, and imagine what it would feel like to be that new you! Take out your journal and write down what you want to achieve, what you want to move toward, and how you are going to do it. Picture yourself with limitless energy and being able to handle your daily tasks and your job while still having enough steam left over for your children and your personal life. How will it feel to put on a swimsuit and feel great about what you see in the mirror? Imagine weighing yourself and loving the number you see! You will start to relish the after-burn of your morning workouts! You have to know and understand what you are moving toward and say good-bye to what you are moving away from to be able to have fitness success and maintain it!

2. Clean out your mental house. Stop putting yourself down! That unfriendly little voice inside your head needs to be silenced now and forever. That super-critical, opinionated alter ego of yours needs to know who the boss is. You are! So what if you gained five pounds on the family vacation cruise? That does not make you a "fat pig." Rather than beating yourself up by complaining, instead compliment yourself by saying something like "Yeah, I did have that chocolate chip cookie for dessert. But I didn't have three of them like I would have done before." You need to learn to stay focused on your objective and stay positive. Don't let the negativity get you down or blur the vision of your destination! Stop whining, and take more control over your actions and your life! Stop playing the victim. It doesn't help you or others around you.

3. Treat yourself with respect. Respect yourself. It's that simple, but we don't do it. If you had a best friend whom you loved with all your might, would you give her a fat-laden, artery-clogging cheeseburger with fries or a crisp and fresh garden salad topped with grilled chicken? Yes, you would give her the salad. But why don't you do this for yourself? Most likely because the psychology behind your actions does not allow you to treat yourself with the respect and consideration you have for those you love. You are self-sacrificing, always giving to others but not to yourself.

Think about this: Your mind and body are temples, and you need to treat them as such. Why would you put something dirty and of no value in a sacred and special place? Well, of course you wouldn't! So start respecting yourself and treating yourself right. You deserve better than processed fast food with little to no nutrients. Also, you deserve to chisel out at least fifty minutes every other day for a weight-training session with a touch of cardio at the end. Remember, you are the most important person in your life. If you can't help yourself, then how can you help others? It all begins with you!

4. Be Creative. What do I mean by "be creative"? I don't mean that you need to be an artist or a philosophical thinker. But we are in this for the long run. Being healthy is a process, a journey, not a one-time event. Fitness and health are going to be your new lifestyle. Therefore, we need to make it fun, full of variety, and interesting.

Ask yourself, "What are my favorite foods and the exercises I love to do most?" If you answered Italian food, then buy a low-fat, low-carb Italian cookbook and learn how to remake your old favorites! And if you love to play tennis, join a tennis club or hire an instructor who will help you strengthen your backhand or give you a better edge on your game. If you love nachos, be creative and reinvent the recipe using low-fat ingredients rather than the real stuff. Just open your mind to new and different tools, and use them as a bag of tricks that will help you fight the war on fat. By being creative, you will make it fun, refreshing, and interesting. You will never experience a dull moment in your new healthy life.

5. Put fitness first. Well, not exactly first, but make it a top priority. It should be a rock in your life. If your car breaks down, exercise. If you get a job promotion, exercise. If your husband leaves you, exercise. No matter what happens—stick to your routine!

Of course, all of us will have bad days and get off of our diets—but refocus yourself, look at your compass, and get back on track! And prepare to be tempted. The strategy of "thinking five steps ahead" will allow you to win at the game of fat loss. You know that you have to attend your family's barbeque dinner with nonstop servings of hot dogs, potato salad, and sugary desserts. So be smart and execute your fitness plan: Munch on a crispy apple before the barbecue; this will fill you up, cutting the edge off of any uncontrollable hunger pangs that might set in while you are there. Then opt for the grilled chicken breast with no bun, a side salad, and an ear of corn with no butter. You can put fitness first and still enjoy your family's social activities without sabotaging your fitness goals!

6. Set yourself up for success. Put health on the shelf and the gym bag in the car! Stock your fridge and pantry with the latest guilt-free snacks and treats. Low-carb and low-fat foods are tasting better and better. Try something new today. Have your gym bag ready to go in the car for a pre- or post-workday workout. Throw in a towel and a change of clothes, and you will have no excuse to skip the gym. Buy used exercise DVDs for little to nothing online and have them ready to go in your family room. Have your running shoes right by the bed so that all you have to do is roll out of the sack into your morning run! Everywhere you go and no matter where you are, your healthy habits will follow you. Therefore, it will be almost impossible to keep from sticking to your plans and reaching your goals.

7. Use your pain to motivate you. Yes, pain *can* be your friend! Use it to your advantage as a tool to motivate you to make a positive change in your life. I said that my technique for losing the fat and getting in shape would be painful—well, almost! I created my success by constantly reminding myself of what I looked like before and the pain I experienced when I was at my heaviest. Get some leverage on yourself. First, it is absolutely necessary for you to take a "before" picture of yourself. Second, it would be best if you put this "before" picture in a place where you can occasionally see it when you need to feel the "pain" and frustration associated with that picture to get you motivated. When you feel your motivation and desire weakening, glance at the picture and remind yourself of the despair you felt when you were at your unhealthiest. To make yourself take action, you have to be at the threshold of pain, looking directly at it. This is where your power and supremacy over your future decisions will come from. Pain will be your friend because you will learn how to manipulate it and use it to your advantage. The pain that I revisited often was surrounded by my overweight "before" photo. I deliberately glanced at my "before" image to use it as my pain, and that coerced me into taking positive action.

This pain was the vital vehicle that propelled me into fast-forward mode, making sure I never pushed the "rewind" button. I used the pain of feeling overweight, frumpy, and not being able to wear the beautiful clothes I wanted to as a therapeutic medium to move me toward my goals. These were the methods that led me to my weight-loss achievements. Please use these techniques to stay on the right path. They are as follows:

- Look at your "before" picture.
- Remember how you felt carrying all that extra weight around.
- Remember how you were treated differently when you were heavier.
- Remember the confidence you started to experience when you felt stronger.
- Compare your old lifestyle with your new, improved one and focus on how great it feels to be healthy!
- And, as I speak from experience, I can't say it enough, but it is necessary to stop playing the victim and start making those improvements in your life now to become victorious!

CHAPTER 3

The Philosophy behind Crack the Code™ and How to Understand It

Crarck the Code™ is based on the principle that muscle tissue burns more calories than fat tissue, therefore increasing metabolism. When your metabolism is increased, it makes it easier to burn fat and keep it off forever. To gain muscle, you must strength-train, provide the growing muscle with sufficient protein, and rest. While "cracking the code" toward your fitness potential, you will learn to love yourself through a positive reward system that is *not* based on food.

Ask any doctor, cardiologist, personal trainer, or licensed nutritionist why some people burn off fat more quickly than others. The unanimous answer is their metabolism! Metabolism can be defined as the rate at which we burn off calories. Our metabolism rate is, unfortunately, inherited. However, fortunately enough, this is where my **Crack the Code™** fat-blasting principles will help you increase your metabolism and lose weight. I will give you the necessary tools and steps to actually stoke your metabolism, turning your body into a roaring furnace that burns off the fat, even when your body is at rest. Taking these steps, in combination with healthy habits in general, will allow you to finally **Crack the Code™** and unlock your weight-loss and fat-burning potential. Congratulations on taking control of your life!

Once you begin my **Crack the Code™** program, you will experience an "aha!" moment. You will realize what it takes for your body to release the fat you have been storing for years. Losing weight only to gain it back and constantly seeing the number yo-yoing up and down on the scale made me feel like a hacker who sits at a computer for hours, days, or maybe even weeks, attempting to hack into a protected site. How frustrated I got! I tried all the fad diets and exercise gadgets. I looked in my closet and found clothes ranging from size zero to size sixteen. I said to myself, "This can't be right!" I looked in my bathroom and saw three scales, a fat measurer, a tape measurer, and a mirror where I would judge my appearance daily. Then, I looked in my bedroom and found the same scenario: weights, an elliptical machine, a jump rope, and the latest, hottest weight-loss gadgets—you name it, I had it. Did all these gizmos work? No! My weight still went up and down!

But remember, from chaotic events in our life come great things. I kept on working at my body, trying to find the right method to do three simple things: lose fat, gain muscle, and increase my energy level. I am proud to say that I did it, and now it is my turn to give you the same tools to help you achieve these same weight-loss results!

My simple plan contains no Band-Aid approaches. I take you straight to the root cause of why some people store fat and some people burn it off by just sitting at their desks. *The key is their metabolism!* I would like to introduce you to a proven way to increase your metabolism right off the bat. The answer is this: You must increase your lean muscle mass. I'm not going to waste your time. It is simple math. To add muscle, you must follow this tried-and-true weight-loss success formula: Weight-train and then fuel the growing muscle with a proper, nutritious food plan that is based on moderate to high levels of protein, fiber-rich carbs, and good-for-you fats!

There are no "diet cards," no "phases," no "steps" and no "for two weeks do this, and for two weeks do that" stages. I'm going to keep it simple, short, and sweet. You will find only good, solid, proven information in CTC that will be transformed into power in your life. A lot of the latest popular diets instruct you to cut out fruit. Fruit in the **Crack the Code™** program is a powerful super-food that is essential. How could the top fitness experts tell you not to eat fruit for two weeks? How misleading! As a specialist in sports nutrition, I would never ask you to do something so ridiculous, harmful, and unsafe. Of course, if you don't eat sweets or have alcohol during the first two weeks of any diet, you will lose weight. That is not rocket science, and you don't need to be a doctor to know that. In the **Crack the Code™** program, I show you not only how to get the number on the scale down but also to keep it down forever while you gain strength and increase the energy in your body! You will also improve the look and feel of your body, inside and out.

Exercise is mandatory in CTC! Some of the top-selling diet books state that exercise is up to you to choose and that it is nonessential to losing weight. What a lie! I have even read a top-selling book written by a cardiologist who stated that exercise is a choice, not a solid part of cardiovascular wellness and physical fitness. Where did he get his degree from? Medical research will show you that all forms of exercise, whether a brisk walk or a super-duper power-pump session in the gym, are beneficial to the cardiovascular system and for the entire body.

I am telling you that you *must* treat exercise in this program like an important business meeting with your body that you cannot be late to or miss. Exercise is just "one of the sequence of numbers" that will help you Crack the Code. There will be no codependency on group meetings, no weekly gatherings, and you won't have to buy any pre-made and pre-processed food. Furthermore, you will not have to slave away in your kitchen finely shredding orange peel and peeling/deseeding/slicing papaya for your next "Chicken Raspberry Spinach Salad." This is definitely not the case with **Crack the Code™**. My book is for the everyday busy person who multitasks. Now, with my codes to fitness success, you will be able to get maximum results with small but smart amounts of effort! You will see maximum results in minimum time.

After reading this fit-lifestyle guide, you will be able to do the following:

- Know how to increase your metabolism with my simple tips and tools.
- Understand the three F's that equal an A+ in weight training.
- Exercise smarter, not harder.
- Understand why weight training is an underestimated lifesaver.
- Know my favorite fundamental weight-training exercises.
- Learn the difference between good and bad carbs and fats.
- Learn why exercising in the morning is the best choice.
- Understand that fitness must start in your mind.
- Learn how fiber is your best friend when it comes to weight loss.
- Learn how to keep from getting bored or discouraged when you hit a plateau.
- Break through mental and physical barriers that keep you from achieving your goals.

CHAPTER 4

Section 1: Ten Basic Principles to Crack the Code™

Let's get ready now to study the core of the **Crack the Code™** principles so that you can stoke your metabolism and start blasting the fat off before you know it! These basic principles will soon become part of your daily healthy lifestyle.

The Ten Basic Principles to cracking the code are as follows:

1. **Eat frequently.**
2. **Exercise in the morning.**
3. **Have a tea party! Drink green tea, and learn how it speeds up your metabolism.**
4. **Lift weights, and the fat will fall! The three F's that equal an A+ in weight training are form, focus, and full range of motion.**
5. **Circuit-train.**
6. **Eat foods high in protein.**
7. **Train in the range of your target heart rate—not under or over.**
8. **Don't overtrain.**
9. **Rest.**
10. **Don't hit a plateau—keep your body guessing.**

Section 2: The Core to Crack the Code™: Easy Steps to Jolt Your Metabolism and Burn Off Fat Efficiently and Effectively

Breakfast

As you begin practicing healthy lifestyle habits, I cannot stress enough the importance of eating breakfast. Consume most of your calories at the beginning of the day or during the middle of the day. "Eat breakfast like a king, lunch like a prince, and dinner like a pauper!" Breakfast is the most important meal of the day. It should also be your largest and most filling meal. When you have a large load of calories in the morning, you will eat less at night, helping you fight off those extra pounds that creep up from late-night eating. And your body will function more effectively and efficiently when fueled in the morning from your nightlong fast. These calories will work with your body to get you up and feeling fully charged for the day, thus thwarting any midmorning hunger pangs.

A weight-loss client of mine, Laura from Arizona, would argue that she was saving calories by not eating breakfast. I took a look at her food log, and it told me what I had feared and expected: She was so ravenous by lunch that she would eat enough for three people! I showed her how she overate and made poor food choices for lunch because her body was crying out for food. She wasn't a "breakfast person," but I convinced her that it was necessary to try eating a balanced meal of protein and good-for-you carbs and fats in the morning. The results spoke for themselves. She had more energy in the morning and ate less at night, and her hunger died down, allowing her to be in more control. She still thanks me to this day for helping her retrain her eating habits so that she eats breakfast in the morning and spreads the calories throughout the day.

When it comes to the best way to eat throughout the day, you'll want to follow these tips:

- Aim to consume five to six mini-meals a day. You need to reward yourself with a constant, even flow of calories that will keep you fueled all day long.
- Aim to have a balance of protein and good-for-you carbs and fats in each meal or snack you consume.

Exercise in the Morning

Don't get me wrong: Any exercise at any time of the day is great. But to get the maximum potential out of any exercise routine, it is absolutely essential that you do your exercise in the morning. I am living proof that anyone can retrain herself to wake up earlier and get in on this early-morning exercise session. I was never a morning person; I often slept in late and went to bed late. This late-to-bed and late-to-rise habit was in direct correlation with the way my body hoarded all that extra weight for so long!

I'm here to tell you that I changed my sleep habits, and so can you. Some mornings will be hard, but you just have to stick to it. You can do it! If not now, then when? Set your alarm at least forty minutes earlier, get your workout clothes ready the night before, and decide what type of exercises you are going to do so there is no last-minute guesswork. Just jump out of bed and begin jump-starting your metabolism! And believe me, you will start to enjoy waking up early in the morning while everyone is still sleeping. (This time will become your special time devoted to you and just you.) You will get hooked and actually look forward to that alarm going off in the morning, reminding you that it is time to give back to yourself with a rewarding dose of good, old-fashioned exercise. Gyms open early especially for early birds and even provide hot coffee and group exercise classes with peppy instructors to get your engine revved for the day ahead!

Here are the benefits of making the morning your choice time to exercise:

- It revs up your metabolism for the entire day.
- It helps set your biorhythm for the day.
- It helps you sleep better at night.
- It increases your energy level throughout the day, giving you a better sense of control.
- You will continue to burn calories throughout the rest of the day—like exercising without even trying.
- It provides you with a better outlook on the day ahead.
- It will make you feel refreshed and ready for anything to come your way.
- It helps you avoid after-work crowds at the gym.
- It kick-starts your metabolism: When you exercise early in the morning, it jump-starts your metabolism and keeps it elevated for hours, sometimes for the rest of the day. That means you're burning more calories all day long just because you exercised in the morning!
- It controls your appetite: Morning exercisers vouch that their appetites are suppressed or regulated for the day and that they aren't as hungry. This allows them to make better food choices. Morning exercise is like a natural appetite suppressant without having to take a pill! Several people have told me that it puts them in a "healthy mindset."
- It increases mental acuity for four to ten hours after exercise (no sense in wasting that while you're sleeping).

Consistency is the cornerstone to success! If you train yourself to exercise first thing in the morning, it is more likely that you will stick with it over the years and build a foundation of success. If you exercise at about the same time every morning and wake up at about the same time on a regular basis, your body's endocrine system and circadian rhythms adjust to that, and physiologically, some wonderful things happen. A couple of hours before you awaken, your body begins to prepare for waking and exercise because it "knows" it's about to happen. Why? Because it "knows" you do the same thing nearly every day.

It is also *much* easier to wake up. When you wake up at different times every day, it confuses your body, which is never really "prepared" to awaken. Set your alarm clock so you wake up at the same time every morning. Even on the weekends! This will train your body and mind to get your optimal rest at night so that you can be your most productive during the day. In addition, your metabolism and all the hormones involved in activity and exercise begin to elevate while you're sleeping, regulating blood pressure, heart rate, and blood flow to the muscles. You'll feel more alert, energized, and ready to exercise when you do wake up.

Setting an appointed time to exercise every morning will become something you look forward to. You are doing something good for yourself by setting aside time to take care of your body and mind. Many find that it's a great time to think clearly, pray, plan their day, or just relax mentally. It is an all-in-one therapeutic session that is free, with countless benefits! And exercising first thing in the morning is the only way to ensure that something else won't crowd exercise out of your schedule. When your days get hectic, exercise usually takes a back seat.

Some mornings, you may be able to fit in only a ten-minute walk, but it's important to try to do something every morning. If finding time to exercise is difficult, you can get up thirty to sixty minutes earlier to exercise (if it's a priority in your life). If necessary, try to go to sleep a little earlier. Also, research has demonstrated that people who exercise on a regular basis have a higher quality of sleep and thus require less sleep.

Maintain Your Target Heart Rate
It is very important that you maintain your target heart rate when you exercise. To receive the full benefits of exercise, you need to pace yourself. When beginning an exercise regimen, it is important to find out what your initial target rate is so that you can determine your fitness level and track your progress.

Your target heart rate should stay between 50 and 85 percent of your maximum heart rate. If you do not have a heart-rate monitor, you may use the "conversational" monitor:

- If you are able to hold a conversation and walk or exercise at the same time, you aren't working too hard.
- If you are able to hold a tune or sing, you are most likely not working hard enough.
- If you get out of breath quickly and have to stop to catch your breath, you are working too hard.

Have a Tea Party!
Although green tea has a moderate amount of caffeine in its chemical makeup, studies show that an interaction occurs between its active ingredients that promotes increased metabolism and fat oxidation. Green tea extract has substantial implications for weight control, especially when taken during the daytime. A person taking green tea extract will increase his or her energy level by 4 percent during a twenty-four-hour period. Because thermogenesis (the rate at which the body is able to burn calories) contributes to 8 to 10 percent of the daily energy expenditure in a typical person, this 4 percent increase due to green tea translates into a 35 to 43 percent increase in daytime thermogenesis.

In addition, green tea extract does not raise the heart rate and blood pressure the way prescription drugs for obesity, like ephedra, do. Green tea also does not overstimulate your adrenal glands like other prescriptions drugs for obesity do.

The best way to incorporate green tea into your weight-loss/fitness regimen is to purchase a well-known brand of organic green tea that contains 150 to 200 milligrams of antioxidants. You can purchase this tea at most grocery and health-food stores. Start by either taking green tea extract in a supplemental form or by drinking a cup of tea every day. Plan to drink green tea with meals to increase your metabolism even more as you eat.

The Benefits of Circuit Training: Blast through Those Plateaus

Let's face it: Plateaus can happen. It's important to remember that if you have faithfully established healthy food and exercise habits as a part of your lifestyle, you can and will attain your fitness goals.

Still, it is important to add circuit training in combination with strength training to reach your weight-loss and fitness potential. This will add an entirely new dimension to your current fitness program. Circuit training allows you to keep your body guessing by adding cardio sprints (ten- to fifteen-minute sessions) intertwined with strength/weight-training moves.

How to Avoid Overtraining

A successful weight-lifting regimen is based on the notion that to build muscle and increase strength, it is necessary to raise your resistance or overload progressively. Muscles must be given adequate time to recover and rebuild so new muscle can form. You can achieve progressive resistance or overloading simply by doing more reps on a set with the same weight. Also, in addition to adding more weight to your reps, you can add progressive resistance by decreasing the amount of time you rest between sets.

It is important to never get too comfortable. To make great gains toward building muscle, you must strive to do more. Your training sessions should get harder and more intense. However, when you make your workouts more intense and harder, it is important that you get enough rest between workouts and allow enough recovery time for your muscles. If this does not occur, you will end up overtraining your muscles. Your overworked muscles will not get bigger but will instead get smaller and weaker. They can tear or become permanently damaged without proper recovery time.

When training intensely, it's very important to take time off from your workouts. You should consider taking a week to ten days off every four to eight weeks to keep your mind and body fresh.

Rest

No, I am not telling you to take a five-hour relaxation session! What I am emphasizing here is that "Rome was not built in a day." Don't be like a flash in a pan with your exercise and food plan. Instead, it is best to function like a fire that gets stronger with every twig and branch that is put on top of it. Fitness is *not* an event but rather a process. Sure, we all will have off days, but we must not lose track of our objective. Keep your eye on the prize, and aim to attain it slowly! Allow yourself a break. I have seen it too many times in the fitness industry: People come in with a lot of drive and heat, and then they soon fizzle out!

Pace yourself. Do not train more than six days a week. I don't train more than four days a week, and people look at me in amazement when they hear this! It is because I have "cracked the code" on my metabolism, which has allowed me to spend less time in the gym and more time with my family, friends, and career. It has given me a quality of life that is limitless! I am not a slave to my exercise and food plans. Rather, they are obedient to me, and I have the upper hand, allowing myself to burn calories more efficiently and effectively because I train and eat smarter, *not harder*! Give yourself the gift of time to keep your eye on the prize; allow your body down time to heal and regenerate the muscle tissue that you are now causing to grow.

Reward

This is the fun section. And I am going to set the record straight: Do not reward yourself with food! Some best-selling diet books out there are brainwashing people to believe that it's all right to reward yourself with chocolate or a sugary sweet for being good. Let's focus on what this is subconsciously telling your mind and body! The same garbage that got us into this overweight and unhealthy situation in the first place is now prized as a reward. How ridiculous! To encourage someone trying to establish a healthy lifestyle to carry Reese's Pieces in her purse as a reward encourages self-sabotaging practices.

Instead, indulge in a hot bath, a trip to the spa or salon, or the favorite pair of skinny jeans you have been dying to wear! Also, treat yourself by buying a package of yoga classes or spinning classes. This is a great idea because at the same time you treat and spoil yourself, you are also setting yourself up for success by purchasing classes that you must use because you spent good money on them. There are so many ways to reward yourself for sticking to your goals and giving yourself the most gorgeous work of art—the body you have always desired.

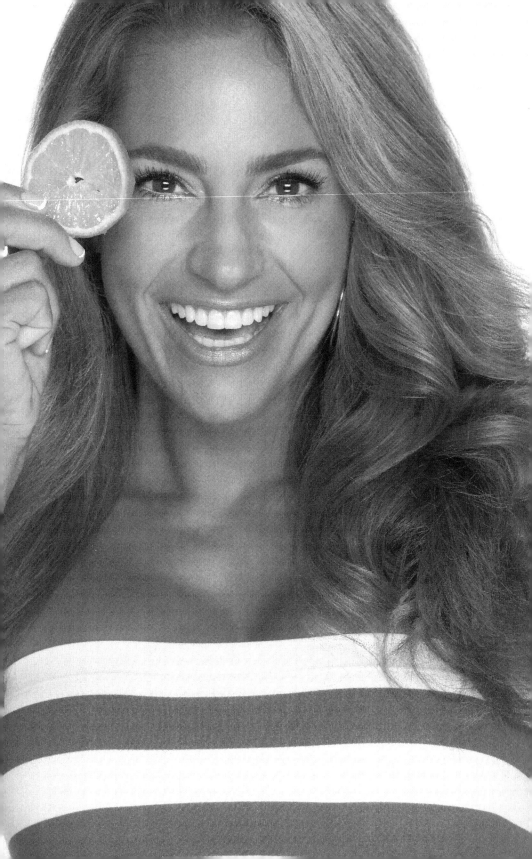

PART TWO:

Stop Eating Accidentally!
The Crack the Code™ Food Plan

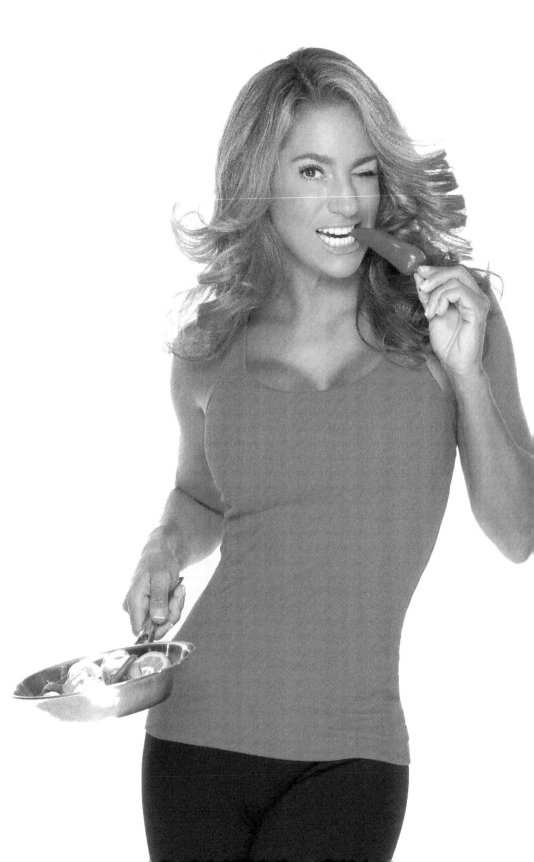

CHAPTER 5

Section 1: Exposing the Truth behind the Latest Fad D-I-E-ts

I hate diets, and you probably do, too. If you look at the first three letters of "diet," what does it spell? D-I-E! But we don't want to *die;* we want to live, and live optimally!

I would like to enlighten you about the various fad diets you may have been exposed to. Through my own trial and error, I have composed a list of *truths* that will dispel the myths behind these diets that not only put your health at risk but also fail to give you the results you need.

Atkins: Meat, meat, and more meat. Yuck is all I have to say! And I'm not the only one with such a harsh reaction to this bizarre diet. It has been dubbed the Nightmare Diet because, yes, you may lose weight, but you do so at the risk of your health and even your life. Even the president of the American College of Nutrition said this has to be the most dangerous diet if followed for any length of time. Former US Surgeon General C. Everett Koop wrote that the Atkins Diet is unhealthy and can be dangerous. With this diet, you are brainwashed into believing that gorging on bacon, heavy cream, and butter, while shunning apples and other nutritious foods, is a sound way to lose weight. It is no wonder, then, that a vast majority of dietary experts have lashed out at the late Dr. Robert Atkins.

Most prestigious scientific bodies in the United States, such as the National Academy of Sciences, join with the American Medical Association and the American Diabetes Association in opposing the Atkins Diet. So do the American Cancer Society, the American Heart Association, the Cleveland Clinic, Johns Hopkins University, the American Kidney Fund, the American College of Sports Medicine, and the National Institutes of Health. In fact, there does not seem to be a single major government or nonprofit medical, nutritional, or scientifically based organization in the world that supports the Atkins Diet. So why should you? As a 2004 medical journal review concluded, the Atkins Diet "runs counter to all the current evidence-based [studies on] dietary recommendations."

The Zone Diet: This impractical diet clutters your mind with its various phases. Honestly, how many "phases" are there? And do I really need to have my food delivered to me every day for every meal? With these questions, I already feel confused and isolated from the rest of society! Plus, it is costly.

Here are some other negative aspects of the Zone Diet:

- It is complicated, and the instructions are too scientific and wordy.
- It is hard to stay on and follow through, which results in fallout and diet relapse.
- It is faulty because it eliminates some essential vitamins and minerals found in certain foods.
- It is expensive to follow, time-consuming, and inconvenient.

Losing weight is a challenge in itself. Why make it more difficult? With CTC, you are getting to the core of the problem, not wasting time and money getting nowhere fast! With CTC, you will learn how to incorporate a healthy balanced diet and learn effective and efficient exercises you can do in the comfort of your own home or at the gym.

The South Beach Diet°: Dr. Arthur Agatston has a wonderful food plan but fails to outline an exercise program, which should be absolutely essential to any weight-loss regimen. CTC differs from the South Beach Diet because it provides fitness *and* nutritional education; it is also safer because there is no "phasing" period, and exercise is mandatory rather than a choice. With CTC, you are encouraged to start an exercise program that will shed pounds safely and help you maintain a healthy weight. CTC clearly illustrates how to work out smarter and not harder so that you lose weight in an efficient and, most importantly, safe manner.

The Fat Flush° Plan: The Fat Flush plan is a detoxing program focused on cleansing the liver—a good way to start a new food plan. However, we can't function forever on a detoxification ritual. While the Fat Flush plan may be helpful temporarily, CTC empowers you with a long-term plan that gets to the root of why some people store fat easily while others burn it off quickly and efficiently. As we learned earlier, the answer to this question lies in our metabolic rate. The Fat Flush plan does not touch on the notion of an exercise regimen, and that ultimately makes the plan the wrong choice for anyone looking to lose weight the safe and healthy way. CTC focuses on the crucial element to long-term weight-loss, which lies in exercise with an emphasis on weight/strength training.

The 3-Hour Diet: The 3-Hour Diet is based on the concept that you can attain weight loss if you eat every three hours, ultimately losing belly fat first. First of all, there is no real rocket science here. Tell us something we already don't know! There is no such thing as "spot" dieting or "spot-reduction exercising." Jorge Cruz's strategy lacks substance, depth, and logic. He states that you can eat ice cream and chocolate and carry around Reese's Peanut Butter Cups with you to stop bingeing. Come on! If I were told I could do that and still actually lose weight, I would buy into it as well! It is an overweight person's dream to hear all of that and get the false comfort that it is possible to lose weight on this type of diet. But with CTC, I do not feed you these misconceptions, and I educate you with the proper fat-fighting tools so that you will lose weight and keep it off forever. My food and exercise plan is not a trend or a fad that will only be exposed in the end, but a strategy for permanent weight loss with longevity. My book also emphasizes the importance of exercising, a critical element that Jorge's book fails to address.

Winning by Losing: Jillian Michaels takes a "triple threat" approach to losing weight. Her diet plan is composed of balanced oxidizers, Asparagus Frittata, and thirty pages on writing goals. I was already frustrated, confused, and discouraged after the first chapter! When I weighed nearly two hundred pounds, I needed help fast! I did not want to be bogged down with too much information or fancy information. I just needed to know what worked. In CTC, I step up to the plate and make it clear what needs to be done. Increasing your metabolism is the key! And to do this is as easy as one, two, three! First, weight train; second, eat a high-protein and moderate good-for-you carb diet; third, rest and reward yourself! It is a wonderful nonstop cycle with the end result being success!

Section 2: Cheating Happens, but It Doesn't Have to Sabotage You

Elizabeth, a client of mine, would argue that because she had already eaten a piece of cake after lunch, the "food floodgates" were open, and her food plan would go out the window. She would binge the day away, believing that because she already sabotaged her diet with that one piece of cake, the entire rest of the day was a food free-for-all! I instilled in her the philosophy that dieting is not an "all or nothing" proposition.

Another client, Jamie from California, puts it this way:

> The keynote to my losing the weight is simple. I'm learning to not be so all or nothing. If I really want something, I have it, but I make up for it in exercise or I eat really clean after that. My food diary is a must. It allows me to monitor whether or not I'm eating too much or too little. Some people don't realize that if you exercise hard, you have to eat. I find that I have to eat complex carbs before weightlifting or else I'm wasting my time with no strength. And being patient is a daily task. We want instant gratification. With fat loss, it's a gradual peeling of layers. With each layer, some issues in your soul pop up, teaching you that self-love and self-discovery go hand in hand.

Jamie, a proud mother of two children, says that her keynote is "learning to *truly* love myself. When I have peeled away all the layers that I want, I will be a new woman." Jamie is an inspiration to us all. She takes it day by day and is patient with herself. She is learning that the key to weight loss is self-love! Eating all day and bingeing is not self-love but the direct opposite.

And what do you do if you ate that extra piece of pie or indulged a little too much? You simply keep your eye on the prize and pick up right where you left off! Eat healthy again, admit that you can do better, exercise, and aim not to repeat the cycle.

Cheat Meals?

As a professional in the fitness industry, I am often asked if I enjoy a cheat meal or a cheat day. My answer is based on wisdom, common sense, reason, and logic. If I have the mindset that I am starving myself from the get-go, I will not get results. I am eating to live, not living to eat. I don't designate a day of the week just to binge by eating whatever I want and how much I want of it! Instead, I am reasonable, balanced, and focused with my food plan. Having two toddler boys around all the time is great for my willpower! I am constantly bombarded with Oreos, mac and cheese, pizza, hot dogs, chicken nuggets, and French fries. But instead of a "cheat meal" in which I could easily consume more than one thousand calories (Fettuccini Alfredo, anyone?), I savor a "cheat bite." Sometimes the small nibble from my son's chocolate chip cookie is just as satisfying as, if not more than, eating the whole thing! I get to enjoy the small taste and the aroma of the cookie without having to work out twice as hard to burn off all those extra calories from the cookie.

Taking "cheat bites" really helps when you are at dinner parties or work functions where everyone else is eating and you don't want to look or feel left out. Simply take your piece of key lime pie, eat one bite, and then leave the rest! Believe me, you will feel so good and proud of yourself when you are looking back at that plate with the almost-entire piece of uneaten pie and all the unnecessary calories that you saved by not eating the whole piece.

Section 3: Super Power Foods and Foods You Should Always Have in Your House

Super-foods are the best bang for your buck and your body! They supersede normal healthy foods because they are chock full of fat-blasting fiber, cancer-fighting antioxidants that fight off free radicals, and are full of healthy vitamins and minerals! Make sure you stock your home's pantry and fridge with these super-foods to give you a super-fit body! One great feature about the JNL Crack the Code™ diet is that you have to eat in order to be healthy, feed sexy and lean muscle tone, and blast off ugly fat!

Breakfast

- Egg-white omelet with veggies and low-fat cheese with a side of whole-wheat toast
- Low-fat milk fruit smoothie blended with protein powder mix and fruit of your choice (My favorite combinations are strawberry–blueberry and banana–peanut butter.)
- Smoked salmon and low-fat cream cheese on a small whole-wheat bagel

Body-Rewarding Snacks

- Apple with two tablespoons of peanut butter
- Low-fat, low-sugar yogurt
- Low-fat string cheese with a side of sliced tomatoes drizzled with olive oil and salt-free Italian seasoning
- Nutritional shake

Lunch

- Grilled chicken salad with a small, whole-wheat roll or whole-wheat crackers
- Blackened salmon with a side of steamed vegetables and brown rice
- Tuna-fish salad made with a touch of low-fat or fat-free mayonnaise on a bed of fresh, crisp greens with side of whole-wheat crackers or whole-wheat roll

Afternoon Snack (4 o'clock or so)

- Handful of almonds (about twelve) and a pear
- Banana sliced lengthwise, smeared with two tablespoons of peanut or almond butter, drizzled with honey and accompanied by a handful of wheat crackers
- Low-fat cottage cheese with a dollop of sugar-free preserves

Dinner
- Baked tilapia with sweet potato and side salad
- Seared Asian seasoned tuna with a side of seaweed salad and miso soup
- Grilled flank steak, sautéed tomatoes, and brown rice with a small side salad

Healthy Fast-Food Choices
We all work and have busy lives with overbooked schedules and demands we cannot keep up with. We simply don't have time to julienne red pepper, mince garlic, and defrost chicken! Let's face it: Although cooking and preparing meals does have certain bonuses, we can't do it every day. So, when we are out in the real world, what do we eat?

With my foolproof list of dos and don'ts and what to look for and what to avoid, eating out or eating on the go is a cinch!

What to Avoid
- Fried foods
- Foods loaded with gravies or heavy sauces
- Sugary treats disguised as healthy foods (granola bars, "snack mix," breakfast bars, etc.)
- Sodas, colas, drinks that pack a whopping 200 calories per serving
- White-bread sandwiches
- Mayonnaise, oil, butter, margarine

What to Buy
- Baked or grilled meats
- Whole-wheat bread or brown rice as a side
- Fresh vegetables and fruits
- Low-fat, snack-size servings that are low in sugar (Read the labels! You can't assume it is healthy just because the word "healthy" appears on the label.)

- Low-sodium alternatives
- Olive oil and flaxseed oil

What to Do

- Always ask for no cheese, no sour cream, or no soy sauce on the food you order. (They are loaded with unnecessary fats or sodium.)
- Always ask for sauce on the side.
- Always request whole-wheat or whole-grain bread when given a choice.
- Choose low-fat milk or skim milk instead of half and half.
- Ask for grilled instead of fried meat or fish.
- Ask for water instead of the diet soda or cola that comes with your meal combo.
- Ask for olive oil instead of butter for your whole-wheat bread.

**BONUS MATERIAL

The Crack the Code™ Grocery List

Proteins

- Boneless, skinless chicken breast
- Tuna (water-packed)
- Fish (salmon, sea bass, halibut)
- Shrimp
- Extra-lean ground beef or ground round (92–96 percent lean)
- Protein powder
- Egg whites or eggs
- Rib-eye steaks or roast
- Top round steaks or roast (aka stew meat, London broil, stir-fry)
- Top sirloin (aka sirloin top butt)
- Beef tenderloin (aka filet, filet mignon)
- Top loin (NY strip steak)
- Flank steak (stir-fry, fajita)
- Eye of round (cube meat, stew meat, bottom round, 96 percent lean ground round)
- Ground turkey, turkey breast slices or cutlets (fresh meat, not deli cuts)

Complex Carbs

- Oatmeal (old-fashioned or quick oats)
- Sweet potatoes (yams)
- Beans (pinto, black, kidney)
- Oat-bran cereal
- Brown rice
- Farina (Cream of Wheat)
- Multigrain hot cereal

- Pasta
- Rice (white, jasmine, basmati, Arborio, wild)
- Potatoes (red, baking, new)

Fibrous Carbs
- Green, leafy lettuce (green leaf, red leaf, romaine)
- Broccoli
- Asparagus
- String beans
- Spinach
- Bell peppers
- Brussels sprouts
- Cauliflower
- Celery

Other Produce and Fruits
- Cucumber
- Banana peppers
- Onions
- Garlic
- Tomatoes
- Zucchini
- Fruit: bananas, apples, grapefruit, peaches, strawberries, blueber-ries, raspberries
- Lemons or limes

Healthy Fats
- Natural-style peanut butter
- Olive oil or safflower oil
- Nuts (peanuts, almonds)
- Flaxseed oil

Dairy and Eggs

- Low-fat cottage cheese
- Eggs
- Low-fat or nonfat milk

Beverages

- Bottled water
- Crystal Light
- Green tea
- Pomegranate juice

Condiments and Miscellaneous

- Fat-free mayonnaise
- Reduced-sodium soy sauce
- Reduced-sodium teriyaki sauce
- Balsamic vinegar
- Salsa
- Chili powder
- Mrs. Dash
- Steak sauce
- Sugar-free maple syrup
- Chili paste
- Mustard
- Extracts (vanilla, almond, etc.)
- Low-sodium beef or chicken broth
- Plain or reduced-sodium tomatoes sauce, puree, paste

CHAPTER 6

Section 1: You Can Just Taste the Goodness: The Crack the Code™ Sample Menu

To make your life easier, here is a sample two-day menu as well as a holiday meal to prepare for a special occasion. My recipes use my super metabolism-boosting foods and ingredients to make for an interesting, creative, and never-boring way to eat healthy!

Day One
Breakfast: Southwest Veggie Omelet Made with Coconut Oil
Serves 1–2

Ingredients:
- 1 tablespoon virgin coconut oil
- 3/4 cups of your favorite veggies suitable for an omelet (I suggest fresh spinach, mushrooms, and green pepper.)
- Cherry tomatoes cut in half
- 3 egg whites and 1 whole egg
- 1 tablespoon skim milk
- Black pepper
- Cayenne pepper

1. In a small pan, melt the coconut oil. Add the vegetables and sauté until tender.
2. Add the cherry tomatoes; stir and sauté for 2 minutes.
3. While the vegetables are sautéing, beat the eggs with milk in a small bowl. Add black and cayenne pepper to taste.
4. Pour eggs into the pan and scramble lightly.

Serve with a slice of low-carb toast, half a cup of prepared old-fashioned oatmeal, or half a cup of high-fiber cereal. You can top your toast with sugar-free preserves and add some fresh strawberries or blueberries to your cereal.

Midmorning Snack: Vanilla Coconut Protein Shake
Ingredients:
- 1 cup skim milk
- 1 scoop of vanilla protein shake mix
- 1 cup ice (depending on preferred consistency)

Blend and serve.

Lunch: Grapefruit Chicken Salad
Serves 3–4

Ingredients:
- 1 1/2 cups grapefruit segments, cut into bite-size pieces
- 2 cups cooked chicken, diced
- 1/4 cup celery, chopped
- 1 scallion, minced
- 1/4 cup low-fat mayonnaise
- 1/4 cup low-fat plain yogurt
- 1/4 cup fresh parsley, minced
- Dash of celery seed

1. Combine all ingredients and mix thoroughly.
2. Serve on a bed of salad greens and with whole-wheat crackers.

Late-Afternoon Snack: JNL Cayenne Coconut Thai Soup

This delicious soup will hold you over until dinner, and it's been proven that soup fills you up quickly, thus curbing your appetite. Make a whole pot and freeze individual portions. Take this soup with you to work and warm it up in the microwave for a hot, delicious snack that will fill you up without filling you with guilt! And it's a great soup to have if you feel a cold coming on. The cayenne helps to fight off fever, and the coconut oil boosts your immune system. This soup is a great addition to a healthy food plan.

Ingredients:
- 1 teaspoon coconut oil
- 1 clove garlic, chopped
- 4 shallots, chopped
- 2 small, fresh red chili peppers, chopped
- 1 cup red bell pepper, sliced lengthwise
- 1 cup broccoli
- 1 tablespoon lemongrass, chopped
- 2 1/8 cups chicken stock
- 6 ounces lean chicken breast, cut into bite-size chunks
- 1 1/2 cups unsweetened coconut milk
- 1 bunch fresh basil leaves

1. In a medium saucepan, heat oil and butter over low heat.
2. Sauté the garlic, shallots, chilies, red bell pepper, broccoli, and lemongrass in oil until fragrant.
3. Stir in chicken stock, coconut milk, and chicken and bring almost to a boil.
4. Simmer on low heat until chicken is cooked.
5. Add some extra cayenne at this point. Make it as hot and spicy as you like!

Dinner: Grilled Grapefruit Marinated Chicken Breasts with Avocado
Bored with chicken? Not with my recipe!

Ingredients:
- 4 chicken breasts
- 1 pink grapefruit
- 1 navel orange
- 1 lemon
- Lemon–pepper seasoning
- One whole avocado, sliced

1. Marinate four chicken breasts overnight in a mixture of freshly squeezed grapefruit, lemons, and oranges.
2. Sprinkle lemon pepper on marinated breasts.
3. Heat grill.
4. Grill chicken breasts, being careful not to over- or undercook.
5. For garnish, grill four slices of grapefruit.
6. Top chicken breasts with grilled grapefruit slices.
7. Serve with a side of avocado, a side of brown rice, and steamed vegetables or salad to make a complete meal.

Treat or Dessert: Chocolate Pound Cake with Cappuccino Pudding
The power of cocoa is unquestionable. Cocoa has been shown to produce the following health benefits:

- It lowers blood pressure.
- It improves circulation.
- It lowers the death rate from heart disease.
- It improves the function of endothelial cells that line blood vessels.
- It defends against destructive molecules called "free radicals," which trigger cancer, heart disease, and stroke.
- It improves digestion and stimulates the kidneys.
- It is used to treat patients with anemia, kidney stones, and poor appetite.

Aim to use the darkest chocolate available, which is 72 percent cocoa; it can be found at Godiva specialty stores.

Ingredients:
- 1 large, fat-free chocolate pound cake (Entenmann's)
- 1/2 cup extra-dark chocolate (found at Godiva)
- 2 cups light silken tofu
- 1 tablespoon dry instant coffee or espresso
- 1 teaspoon boiling water
- 1/2 cup of low-fat sour cream
- 1/4 cup sugar
- 1/4 cup Splenda
- 1 teaspoon vanilla extract
- 1/2 teaspoon cinnamon

1. Drain tofu and blend in food processor until smooth.
2. Melt the dark chocolate and add to tofu.
3. Combine coffee with boiling water and add tofu.
4. Add sour cream, vanilla, and cinnamon, and blend until creamy.
5. Slice pound cake and place on serving dishes. Add a large dollop of the cappuccino pudding.
6. Garnish with large strawberries and slivered almonds if you choose.

Day 2
Breakfast: Fruit Smoothie with Coconut Oil
Start the day off with a breakfast bang! Wash down your vitamins with a rich, delicious protein smoothie thickened with virgin coconut oil. The main differences between virgin coconut oil and refined coconut oil are the scent and taste. All virgin coconut oils retain the fresh scent and taste of coconuts, while the refined coconut oils have a bland taste due to the refining process.

Ingredients:
- 2–3 tablespoons of virgin coconut oil (at room temperature; it doesn't matter if is it liquid or solid)
- 1 scoop of vanilla whey protein powder
- 1 cup of skim milk
- 3 ice cubes
- Fruit of your choice or whatever you have in the fridge at the time—bananas, blueberries, and strawberries work well.

Place all of the ingredients in a blender or food processor and blend until smooth.

Midmorning Snack: Crack the Code™ Cottage Cheese
Ingredients:
- 1 snack pack of fat-free cottage cheese
- 1 tablespoon sugar-free preserves
- 1 teaspoon coconut oil
- Dash of cinnamon

1. Swirl the sugar-free preserves in with the cottage cheese.
2. Drizzle in coconut oil and add a dash of cinnamon if you like.
3. Accompany your power protein snack with a side of whole-wheat crackers and a cup of hot green tea, or serve it cold if you wish.

Lunch: Siciliano Protein-Packed Antipasto
This dish makes an interesting and fun lunch that is just as pleasing to the eye as it is to the tummy!

On a plate, arrange the following ingredients:
- Lean cuts of turkey breast
- Black and green olives, rinsed off to remove excess salt
- Low-fat or fat-free Swiss cheese
- Low-fat mozzarella cheese

- Cherry tomatoes cut in half and drizzled with virgin olive oil
- Broccoli florets and carrot sticks
- Pickled banana peppers
- Whole-wheat crackers

Late-Afternoon Snack: Coconut Cookies

Approximate yield: 1 dozen

They sound sinful, but they aren't. They're actually great for you because they are low in sugar, they have a high fiber content from the oats, and the flaxseeds add texture and are a great source of essential fatty acids. What a great, guilt-free treat! Add a serving of fat-free, snack-size cottage cheese, and you are set until dinner!

Ingredients:
- 1 cup unsweetened coconut flakes
- 3 tablespoons warm water
- 1 egg
- 1 tablespoon honey
- 1 teaspoon coconut oil (for greasing the cookie sheet)
- 1/4 cup flaxseeds
- 1 cup old-fashioned oats

1. Mix warm water and honey together.
2. Add the coconut flakes.
3. Beat in the egg. Mix thoroughly.
4. Form into balls and drop by spoonful on well-greased cookie sheet.
5. Bake at 400 degrees Fahrenheit for 12–15 minutes.

Dinner: Siciliano (Turkey) Meatballs

One of my favorite memories as a child is sitting around a table enjoying a bowl of spaghetti and meatballs. Now I exchange the high-fat ground beef for low-fat turkey, slashing the calories while keeping the protein high and the taste delicious! As for the pasta, use whole-wheat or spinach pasta to increase the fiber. Yes, you can have carbs, but the right ones. And watch your portion control. Aim for no more than one cup of pasta and four meatballs.

Ingredients:
- 4 slices dry whole-wheat bread
- 1/2 cup water
- 2 tablespoons cold-pressed extra-virgin olive oil
- 4 egg whites
- 3/4 cup low-fat Parmesan cheese
- 1 pound ground turkey
- 1 tablespoon salt
- 2 teaspoons oregano

1. Leave bread out all day so it is dry.
2. Put bread in bowl and pour water over it.
3. Let water soak in.
4. Squeeze out excess water and discard.
5. Break up bread with fingers.
6. Add egg whites, Parmesan cheese, parsley flakes, meat, salt, and oregano.
7. Mix together with your hands.
8. Add salt to taste.
9. Roll into two-inch balls and put on cookie sheet sprayed with non-stick oil. Bake in 350-degree oven for 20–30 minutes.

Treat or Dessert: Grapefruit Tart
Ingredients:
- 2 pink grapefruits
- 1 orange
- 1/2 cup fat-free, sugar-free vanilla pudding
- 8 prebaked sponge cake shells

1. Using a sharp knife, peel rind and pith from grapefruits and orange.
2. Cut into sections, and set them aside to drain.
3. Spread vanilla pudding over a sponge cake shell.
4. Arrange drained grapefruit and orange sections over curd. Serve immediately.

Dessert: Siciliano Tiramisu

This is a super protein-packed dessert loaded with taste, creaminess, and sweetness—all the things a dessert should have but without the guilt! Extra cocoa powder and delicious, tart strawberries add to the antioxidant punch this dessert packs.

Ingredients:
- 1 large container fat-free ricotta cheese
- Cocoa powder
- 5 teaspoons instant espresso powder or instant coffee powder
- 1 teaspoon Splenda or Equal
- 1 teaspoon vanilla extract
- 1 teaspoon almond extract
- Sugar-free/fat-free chocolate pudding
- Slivered roasted almonds
- Ladyfingers
- Fresh cut strawberries
- Fat-free whipped cream

1. In a bowl, mix the ricotta cheese, cocoa powder, almond extract, vanilla extract, and Splenda. Set aside.
2. In a 9" x 9" dessert tray, layer the ingredients as follows: ladyfingers, ricotta mixture, and low-fat, sugar-free chocolate pudding. Top with fat-free whipped cream and garnish with roasted slivered almonds and fresh strawberries.

Special-Occasion Dinner

Starter/Appetizer: Roasted Red Peppers in Olive Oil and Garlic with Grilled Shrimp

Peppers are powerhouses packed with an incredible amount of vitamin C, giving you almost 300 percent of your RDA per serving! Shrimp is an excellent source of low-fat, low-calorie protein that is high in selenium, which is needed in small doses for overall health. And everyone knows the wonders of olive oil and garlic! So start your meal off right with this appetizer.

Ingredients:
- 4 large red bell peppers, cut in half
- Olive oil
- 2 tablespoon fresh basil, minced
- 2 teaspoons balsamic vinegar
- 1 loaf of whole wheat bread, warmed to a light crisp in toaster oven
- Salt-free Italian seasoning
- 1 clove garlic
- 24 pieces of fresh shrimp, peeled and deveined

1. Rub the peppers with olive oil and place on a cookie sheet.
2. Broil on high for 3–5 minutes, until you see the skin bubble up and turn brownish black. Take peppers out and place inside a plastic bag. (This trick will allow you to take the skin off more easily). When the peppers are cool, rub off the skin.
3. Place the "meat" of the peppers in a bowl and add vinegar and seasoning.
4. Serve on a colorful plate with the side of bread, or place the peppers on top of the bread.
5. In a heated skillet, add olive oil and slightly brown the garlic. Add the shrimp, cooking 3–4 minutes until pink.
6. Serve with peppers and bread.

Salad: Barley Vegetable Salad with Feta

Hands down, barley is the best whole grain for you because it contains more fiber than brown rice. One cup of whole-grain barley flour has nearly 15 grams of dietary fiber and just 2 grams of fat. Whole-grain wheat has comparable levels of dietary fiber, but the fiber in wheat is almost entirely insoluble. Barley has a very high level of viscous soluble fiber (called beta-glucan)—about 25 percent of the fiber found in whole-grain barley is water-soluble.

Studies have shown that a diet high in viscous fiber such as beta-glucan helps lower blood LDL cholesterol (the so-called "bad" cholesterol) levels, a risk factor for heart disease. Such diets may also help stabilize blood glucose levels, which could benefit people with non-insulin-dependent diabetes.

Whole-grain barley contains high levels of minerals and important vitamins like calcium, magnesium, phosphorus, potassium, vitamin A, vitamin E, niacin, and folate. The vitamin E found in whole-grain barley contains both tocopherols and tocotrienols—powerful antioxidants that research indicates may reduce the risk of certain cancers and help lower blood pressure.

Barley is usually used in soups or stews, but I like to use it to "beef" up a delicious vegetable salad sprinkled with feta. Dig in!

Ingredients:
- 1 cup barley, cooked and hulled
- 1 cup water
- 1 green bell pepper, seeded and diced
- 1 1/2 cups carrots, chopped
- 1 cup red cabbage
- 1/2 cup red onion, minced
- 1/4 cup sun-dried tomatoes, minced
- 1 tablespoon red wine vinegar
- 2 teaspoons horseradish mustard
- 1 teaspoon olive oil

- Ground pepper to taste
- Dash of cayenne pepper
- 2 tablespoons feta cheese

1. Cook hulled barley per directions. Put in a large mixing bowl; add green pepper, carrots, cabbage, tomatoes, and onion.
2. In a small bowl, mix together vinegar, mustard, and oil.
3. Pour over barley mixture and stir to coat.
4. Top with feta cheese. Season with black and cayenne pepper.

Soup: Spicy Winter Squash

Squash is loaded with vitamin C (great for boosting your immune system and fighting off colds) and fiber (to keep your internal functions working regularly). The cayenne is great for circulation, and the coconut oil has medicinal properties to fight off infections and thyroid overstimulation. But your family won't even think of how good this soup is for them because of how rich and delicious it is!

Ingredients:
- 3/4 Spanish onion
- 2 teaspoons coconut oil
- 2 1/2 teaspoons curry powder
- 1 dash cinnamon
- 1/2 teaspoon cayenne pepper
- 4 cups reduced sodium, nonfat chicken or vegetable broth
- 5 large squashes, baked until soft, then pureed
- 1 sweet potato, baked until semisoft and then cubed
- Black pepper
- Topping: fat-free sour cream and whole-wheat croutons

1. In a large saucepan, sauté onion in oil for 2 minutes.
2. Add curry powder and peppers, stirring to coat.
3. Add broth and sweet potatoes, and bring to a boil.

4. Reduce heat to medium, partially cover, and cook 7–10 minutes.
5. Remove from heat and top with a dollop of sour cream and whole-wheat croutons.

Entrée: Baked Blackened Salmon Steaks with Mango and Black Bean Salsa

Salmon is my favorite fish; it's loaded with omega-3 fat, which is great for our skin and fights off cancer. The only way to get omega-3 fats is to eat them because your body does not make them. The fruit in the salsa adds a kick of sweetness and is loaded with vitamin C. The black beans add fiber and are rich in antioxidants.

Ingredients:
- 1 large mango, pitted and diced into ½-inch pieces (1 1/2 cups)
- 1 kiwi, peeled and diced (1/2 cups)
- 15 ounces black beans, rinsed and drained
- 1/3 cup cilantro, chopped
- 2 scallions, sliced
- 2 teaspoons honey
- 1/2 teaspoon salt
- 1/4 teaspoon cayenne pepper
- 2 tablespoons salt-free blackening seasoning
- 1 lime, squeezed with juice set aside
- 4 salmon steaks, 4 ounces each

1. Heat oven to 350 degrees.
2. Make the salsa: In a mixing bowl, toss the first nine ingredients with half of the lime juice. Set the salsa aside.
3. Place salmon steaks on a cooking tray.
4. Drizzle the remaining lime juice over the fish.
5. Sprinkle both sides with the blackening seasoning.
6. Bake until cooked through, about 15–20 minutes. Top with salsa.

Dessert: Grilled Pears and Peaches with Warm Honey Sauce
While pears and peaches are loaded with fiber, walnuts are loaded with omega-3 fat, and blueberries are an antioxidant powerhouse. It would be sinful *not* to eat this dessert because it is just so good for you!

Ingredients:

Honey Dressing
- 1 cup low-fat vanilla yogurt
- 2 tablespoons honey
- 1 tablespoon fresh lemon juice
- 1 tablespoon coconut oil

Topping
- Chopped walnuts
- Unsweetened coconut flakes
- 1 pint of blueberries, washed
- 1/4 cup chopped fresh mint
- 4 ripe pears
- 4 ripe peaches

1. Preheat oven to 300 degrees.
2. Whisk the yogurt, honey, coconut oil, and lemon juice in a small bowl.
3. In another bowl, combine the blueberries and mint.
4. Place in fridge until ready to use.
5. Lightly brush pears and peaches with coconut oil and grill.
6. Place grilled fruit in mixing bowl with blueberries and mint. Evenly divide among four plates; drizzle with honey sauce and top with walnuts.

**BONUS MATERIAL
Crack the Code™ Protein Shakes

Crack the Code™ Iced Chai Protein Shake
Prep Time: 3 minutes

Ingredients:
- 8 ounces water
- 1 scoop vanilla- or chai-tea-flavored whey protein
- ½ cup chai-tea concentrate
- 1 dash cinnamon
- 1 dash ground ginger
- Orange or cranberry juice

1. Pour water into blender.
2. Add powder, chai-tea concentrate, cinnamon, and ground ginger.
3. Blend on medium speed for 15 seconds.
4. Add orange juice and/or cranberry juice.

JNL Fit Tip: If you cannot locate chai-flavored protein powder, you can use vanilla-flavored powder. You can usually find chai-tea concentrate in the coffee and tea section of your grocery store.

Crack the Code™ Cookies and Cream Protein Shake
Prep Time: 3 minutes

Ingredients:
- 12 ounces cold water
- 1 scoop whey cookies-and-cream-flavored protein powder
- ¼ cup Cool Whip Lite
- 6 ice cubes
- 3 chocolate wafer cookies

1. Pour water into the blender. Add protein powder and blend on medium speed for 15 seconds.
2. Add Cool Whip and ice cubes; blend for 30 seconds on high speed.
3. Add cookies and blend on medium speed until mixed.
4. Pour into a tall glass and enjoy.

Crack the Code™ Chocolate–Peanut Butter Protein Shake
Prep Time: 3 minutes

Ingredients:
- 12 ounces cold water
- 1 packet chocolate whey protein
- 1 tablespoon natural peanut butter
- 6 ice cubes

1. Pour water into blender. Add protein and blend on medium speed for 15 seconds.
2. Add peanut butter and blend for 30 more seconds.
3. Add ice cubes and blend on high speed until smooth (about 30 more seconds).
4. Pour into a tall glass and enjoy.

Section 2: Crack Your Weight-Loss Code with My Favorite Supplements

Listen, we are all super busy and don't have enough time to eat all the food we need in order to be our healthiest! So my Body FX line of nutritional supplements is the most exceptional you can use for optimal health! We also included a Body FX supplement to help curb cravings, and a detox cleanse that you should use first in order to kick start your metabolism! To purchase the entire line of JNL-approved supplements, go to www.Fusion.GetBodyFX.com.

1. Shake FX – Meal Replacement System

Shake FX features our SpectroActive concentrated active ingredient technology. Because it is nearly impossible to put five to nine servings of fruits and vegetables in a single serving of any meal replacement, we use the only true method to get those five to nine servings in our product. Our SpectroActive fruit and vegetable formula concentrates the phytonutrients and antioxidant equivalent of nine servings of fruits and vegetables in every serving. It takes between ten to twenty pounds of fresh vegetables to make just one pound of SpectroActive concentrate.

We also use the SpectroActive technology to create our Adaptogen formula to improve recovery, energy levels, resistance to stress, and for our StayLean formula that promotes fat loss without sacrificing muscle or dehydrating you.

- **Shake FX** does not contain sugar, dextrose, maltodextrin, fructose, or any other sweeteners except for the ideal combination of erythritol and stevia.
- **Shake FX** features our CleanCarb source of antioxidant and nutrient rich carbohydrates from yam powder and pomegranate juice powder.

- **Shake FX** contains our omega fiber, which is a combination of flax and chia seed fiber and contains the valuable and essential omega-3 oils.
- **Shake FX** also contains a prebiotic and probiotic to replenish and feed the beneficial bacteria and improve digestion and elimination.
- **Shake FX** contains a digestive enzyme blend to help you digest and assimilate the high-quality proteins, fats, and carbohydrates in the product.

2. Energy FX – Energy Shot

Our energy product contains a true, microencapsulated, six-hour, time-released source of caffeine. This is a huge breakthrough in energy supplements. By modulating the release of caffeine you don't over-stimulate your adrenal glands and you don't set your metabolism up for a crash.

This slow and deliberate release prevents the jitters and that stressed, nervous feeling common with coffee, energy drinks, and products like 5-hour Energy. Our energy product contains a small amount of natural caffeine from green tea and yerba maté that gives a slight initial boost of energy. Then slowly the true time release begins, giving you all the energy you need for training and your busy life without the downside of crashing and depleting your reserves.

Our energy product also contains threonine, a special amino acid found in green tea, which helps balance the effects of caffeine. This product can be used as a pre-workout supplement or as a needed source of extra energy.

3. After FX – Post-Workout Formula

Our post-workout supplement combines the ProMatrix Plus highly bio-available protein, our CleanCarb for replacing glycogen stores, and a SpectroActive formula to make your hormone-insulin function better for optimal amino acids in your muscle and optimal storage of your muscle fuel, glycogen.

4. Cleanse FX – Fast Start Weight Loss and Detox

This product supports fast initial weight loss through cleansing your body, stabilizing your blood sugars, reducing cravings, and activating fat burning. This product contains a new and highly effective approach to multisystem detoxification.

Our fast start product also contains SpectroActive concentrates designed to help detoxify your liver, bloodstream, lymphatic system, kidneys, small intestine, and large intestine.

Just take the fast start product for two days in place of meals and you will activate your body's fat-burning ability, cleanse your entire body, and get your weight loss off to a motivating start.

5. Slim FX – Weight-Loss Supplement

The biggest challenges of modern day weight loss are the out of control hunger and cravings and unstable blood sugar. We have a solution. It is a combination of three ingredients that helps you feel satisfied, helps eliminate cravings, and literally controls the amount of starch and sugar that reaches your bloodstream.

All you do is take two delicious chewable wafers and some water before a meal and the battle between your mind and your body, craving versus satisfaction, calm versus jittery, and knowing when you've had enough versus eating too much become under your control. And as a result, your ability to lose weight skyrockets, dramatically lowering the stress on your body and mind to improve your quality of life.

6. Protein FX: ProMatrix Plus Protein
Bioavailability Over Six Hours

Bioavailability is the amount of protein available for your body to use over a set period of time. Our blend has a mixture of four protein types: whey protein isolate, micellar casein, whey protein concentrate, and calcium caseinate. The assimilation and utilization rate for each type of protein is unique to its formulation, allowing the body to assimilate and utilize protein over an extended period of time, up to six hours. This staggered protein distribution ensures the optimal supply of amino acids necessary for protein synthesis while keeping protein turnover to a minimum.

Hydrolyzation and Instantization
Hydrolyzation is the process of breaking down protein and removing the lactose, leaving just the protein, minerals, and peptide fractions. Hydrolyzed protein can be absorbed by the body much quicker.

The process of instantizing proteins reduces the particle size and allows for much easier blending and mixing. In short, instantizing reduces the clumping effect when shaking or blending powder.

iG Recovery Proteins
iG recovery proteins have anti-inflammatory properties, help the body initiate defense against pathogens and mutating cells, and help maintain immune homeostasis. Acting as "communicators" between cells, iG proteins help regulate immune, hormonal, and metabolic pathways.

Peptizyme SP
Peptizyme is a systemic enzyme that reduces metabolic inflammation resulting from strenuous exercise. Peptizyme has the ability to break down fibrin, a tough protein arranged in long fibrous chains. Fibrin forms barriers around areas of inflammation such as muscle tissue. Peptizyme breaks these barriers down, allowing healing nutrients to be absorbed into the surrounding tissues.

Protease 1 and 2
Protease 1 and 2 are enzymes that break down protein for digestion. These important enzymes break the peptide bonds in the proteins, liberating the muscle-building amino acids. Protease enzymes also have the ability to digest unwanted debris in the bloodstream, including certain bacteria and viruses.

Glutamine Peptides

Glutamine is a conditionally essential amino acid. The conditions under which glutamine becomes essential to the human body normally occur during exercise. Supplementing with glutamine before, during, and after exercise is critical to maintaining bioavailable levels of glutamine in the body.

Colostrum

Rich in Insulin Growth Factor 1 (IGF-1), colostrum has been shown to increase bone-free lean body mass when supplemented. Colostrum also contains proline-rich polypeptides (PRP), which are small immune signaling peptides that have been shown to reduce the spontaneous or induced mutation in DNA.

Collagen

The most abundant protein in the animal kingdom, collagen is the main component of connective tissue. Our blend contains collagen, not specifically as a nutritive protein source as it is an incomplete protein, but instead to supplement the body with additional collagen. This extra collagen is used as a major component of the endomysium, the layer of connective tissue that sheaths muscle fibers.

Digestive Enzymes

Our blend contains a mixture of digestive enzymes to aid in the breakdown of nutrients by the digestive system. This greatly reduces the bloating and gas issues that some individuals experience when taking a protein supplement. The digestive enzyme matrix in our blend covers all classes of substrates: proteins, fats and fatty acids, carbohydrates (starches and sugars), and nucleic acids.

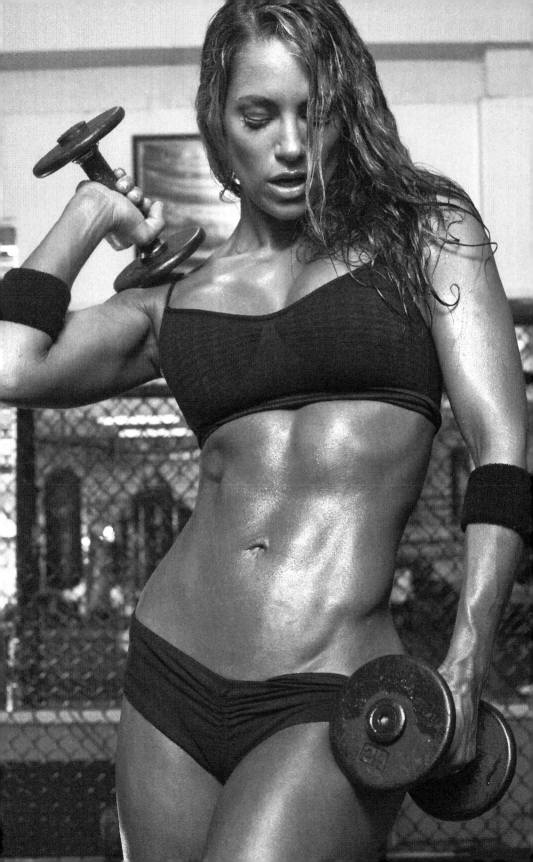

PART THREE:

Exercise Smarter, Not Harder:
Get Maximum Results in Minimum Time

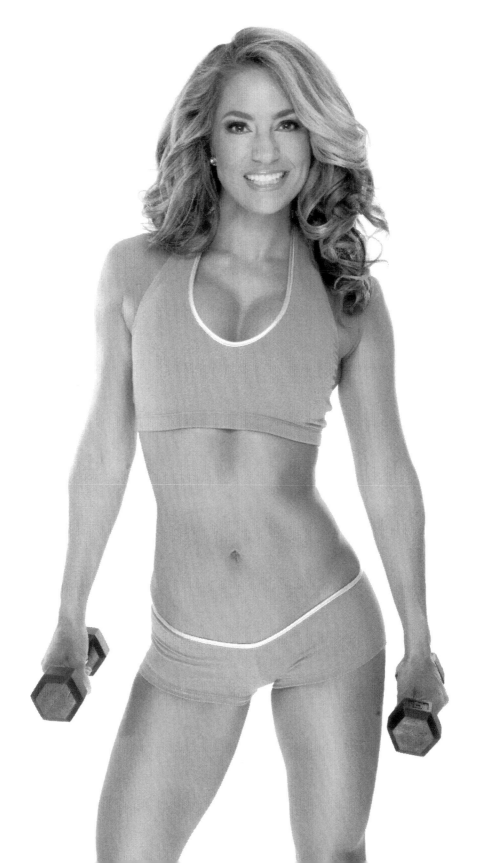

CHAPTER 7

Section 1: Dispel the Myths of Weight Training: Fat Loss for Good

You don't have to be a "muscle head" or a professional weight lifter to enjoy the numerous benefits of incorporating weight training into your exercise regimen. In the long-term scheme of things, weight training actually becomes more important than cardio because it delivers the same benefits as cardio, but you will not get the same benefits of weight training in your cardio workout alone.

Here is a great list of all the advantages of weight training:
- Improves posture.
- Fights off osteoporosis.
- Gives your body shape and tone.
- Increases strength.
- Increases energy.
- Increases confidence.
- Provides an I-can-do-anything attitude that you don't get from just "dancing around" to music in a cardio class.
- Improves your muscular endurance.
- Will *not* develop big muscles on women…just toned muscles.
- Makes you less prone to lower-back injuries.

- Increases your resting blood pressure.
- Decreases your risk of developing adult-onset diabetes.
- Reduces your risk for developing colon cancer.
- Increases your HDL cholesterol (the good type).
- Improves the functioning of your immune system.
- Lowers your resting heart rate, a sign of a more efficient heart.
- Improves your balance and coordination.
- Elevates your mood.

And the most important reason to weight-train is that it boosts your metabolism! How does it do that? The less muscle we have, the lower our metabolic rate. That's why most adults get fatter as they get older. But you'll develop more muscle, boost your metabolism, and actually be able to eat more without gaining weight if you work out with weights two or three times a week.

Section 2: No More Excuses! Empower Yourself by Dispelling the Negativity

In this section, I address some common excuses I have heard—and even believed—about weight training. The responses to those excuses may surprise you.

Excuse #1: I can't build muscle if I don't have any to start with. Answer: We all have muscle, and the time to start building more is now if you have never lifted before.
Remember, what you don't use you will lose. We just naturally grow weaker as we age. We lose up to half a pound of muscle every year after age twenty-five without some kind of regular strength training. With weight training, we stay stronger longer and look better, too.

Excuse #2: But I'm too old to start lifting weights.
Answer: It's never too late to start!

You can boost your strength and improve the way you look and feel no matter how old, weak, or out of shape you are by getting involved with a sensible weight-training program. People over forty or with high blood pressure, heart disease, back pain, arthritis, and other health problems should check with their doctors before beginning any kind of exercise program.

Excuse #3: Weight training is no better than all the other exercises out there.
Answer: Weight training gives you benefits that other exercises just *cannot* deliver on.

In addition, weight training actually helps you to be a better runner, better yogi, and a better Pilates student!

Excuse #4: But weight training won't really increase my metabolism.
Answer: Yes, it does boost your metabolism!

It's a basic equation: The less muscle we have, the lower our metabolic rate. But weight training will help you develop more muscle, boost your metabolism, and eat more without gaining weight.

Excuse #5: Weight training doesn't really give me a better quality of life.
Answer: Yes, it does! You will shed years from your physique and enjoy the confidence and the new sense of inner strength that it gives you.

Building strength can build character. You *will* feel more confident, more in control, and more able to do the kinds of things that make life worthwhile—like carrying your ten-year-old child to playing eighteen holes of golf—when you feel strong. Stronger muscles also can improve your sports performance so you can hit the ball harder, run faster, and jump higher.

Excuse #6: I will only hurt myself from the stress of weight training. Answer: This statement could not be further from the truth. Actually, it is the exact opposite! Weight training gives you greater protection against injury.

The stronger (and more flexible) you are, the less likely you are to suffer injuries that keep you from staying active and having fun.

Excuse #7: Yeah, weight training may strengthen my bones, but all I care about is losing those last five pounds and getting down two more sizes.

Answer: Remember that health isn't about the number on the scale or the size of the clothing you wear.

It is important to understand that by strengthening your bones with weight training, you will experience a better quality of life as you age. Strength training builds bone density, protecting you from certain problems as you age, especially osteoporosis.

CHAPTER 8

Crack the Code™ with These "Perfect Ten" Moves!

J NL Fusion is the hottest and most effective workout to date! It's the workout method that I created out of my need for max results in minimal time and wanting the body and physique of a super fitness model who graces all of the hot fitness magazine covers! The formula of "working smarter, not harder" lies in the simple realization that when you "infuse" your weight training workout with "super spiking cardio bursts," you are burning more calories and thus blasting more fat because your heart rate has already been increased during your weight-training session. This is the power of the JNL Fusion Workout Method! For more info, and to purchase my JNL Fusion exercise DVDs, please visit www.Fusion.GetBodyFX.com.

What makes my JNL Fusion Workout Method so powerful is the fact that it's designed to be user friendly for all fitness levels, from beginner to intermediate to advanced! I focus on the foundation of resistance training, for the benefit of toning sleek and sexy athletic muscles, while burning off ugly fat with my super spiking cardio bursts. To get started right now, I included below the list of my JNL Fusion Perfect 10 Moves! Just pick some exercises from below, and then "infuse" them by adding a thirty-second cardio burst in between your sets!

Lower Body
1. Lunges
2. Squats
3. Inner-thigh plié squats
4. Calf raises
5. Single-leg kickbacks

Upper Body
1. Overhead shoulder press
2. Bicep curls
3. Triceps kickbacks, or triceps overhead press
4. Chest press
5. Bent-over lateral rows

Bonus Moves
- "Whittle your middle" twists
- Butt blasters
- Step-ups

In every field, there are fundamental basics that build a platform of success. We all need to start somewhere. Let's master the foundation of these "Perfect Ten" moves, and then we can add the really fun exercises that make up the last 10 percent of creating a healthy physique that looks incredible, too!

All of these moves can be performed easily in the comfort of your own home with hand weights, or they can be executed in the gym. To make working out easier, invest in a small "personal home gym" that you can store away in the corner of any room you choose to work out in. I suggest a mat for your floor work, three five- to eight-pound hand weights, a stability ball, and an indoor cardio machine such as a stair climber or a NordicTrack.

Lower Body

1. **Lunges:** Put one leg behind you, and then the other, in a slightly open stance to aid your balance. Gently lower and then raise yourself up, focusing on squeezing the glutes, hamstrings, and quads. Perform three sets of eight to twelve reps to build muscle. Perform three sets of eighteen to twenty-one reps to gain muscular endurance and strength.

2. **Squats:** Open your legs in a wide stance, about shoulder width apart. Hold hand weights to add resistance. Gently lower yourself down, bending at the knees; avoid overextending at the knees. (Keep your knees at a 90 degree angle and nothing more.) Keep your abs in tight, with both your chest and chin up. Breathe out as you lower yourself, and breathe in as you come up. Perform three sets of eight to twelve reps to build muscle. Perform three sets of eighteen to twenty-one reps to gain muscular endurance and strength.

3. **Inner-thigh plié squats:** Perform the same way as you did the squats, but turn your toes outward. Perform three sets of eight to twelve reps to build muscle. Perform three sets of eighteen to twenty-one reps to gain muscular endurance and strength.

4. **Calf raises:** Balance on one leg and raise yourself up and down using your calf. Switch legs. Use hand weights for added resistance. Perform three sets of eight to twelve reps to build muscle. Perform three sets of eighteen to twenty-one reps to gain muscular endurance and strength.

5. **Single-leg kickbacks**: Bring one leg back and point your toe. Raise your leg up and down, squeezing your glute region. Switch legs. Use ankle weights for added resistance. Perform three sets of eight to twelve reps to build muscle. Perform three sets of eighteen to twenty-one reps to gain muscular endurance and strength.

Upper Body

1. **Overhead shoulder press:** With abs held in tight, chest up high, and chin up, bring your elbows to a 90 degree angle beside your head. Holding hand weights, gently raise the weights up into a parallel position without the weights touching. Squeeze all the way up and then gently bring the weights back down, not letting your elbows go below a 90 degree angle. Perform three sets of eight to twelve reps to build muscle. Perform three sets of eighteen to twenty-one reps to gain muscular endurance and strength.

2. **Bicep curls:** Bring shoulders up and then down to lock into place. Use a weight that is challenging to you. With your elbows locked in at your sides, bring the weight up and then down, performing this action with both arms at the same time. Perform three sets of eight to twelve reps to build muscle. Perform three sets of eighteen to twenty-one reps to gain muscular endurance and strength.

3. **Triceps kickbacks, or triceps overhead press:** This exercise is great for blasting the flab off the back of your arms! With abs in tight, chin and chest up, and body bent over at the hips, bring your elbows up and back. Then, with a squeezing motion, bring the weights back and then again into starting position. Perform three sets of eight to twelve reps to build muscle. Perform three sets of eighteen to twenty-one reps to gain muscular endurance and strength.

4. **Chest press:** Lying either on the floor or on a bench, while holding dumbbells, bring your elbows to a 90 degree angle and then squeeze up, concentrating on the contraction you feel in your chest muscles. Gently lower your elbows in a slow and controlled manner. Perform three sets of eight to twelve reps to build muscle. Perform three sets of eighteen to twenty-one reps to gain muscular endurance and strength.

5. **Bent-over lateral rows:** With abs held in tight, chest up high, a slight arch in the back, shoulders down, and knees slightly bent, bend over while holding weights that are challenging for you. Bring

the weights up and back, squeezing your back together, and then release. Perform three sets of eight to twelve reps to build muscle. Perform three sets of eighteen to twenty-one reps to gain muscular endurance and strength.

Bonus Moves

- **"Whittle your middle" twists:** With a towel held behind your head, with elbows parallel to the floor, twist at the waist back and forth, focusing on tightening your torso area. Perform three sets of twenty twists.
- **Butt blasters:** This is great if you're looking for an instant booty lift! Simply lie on the floor, stomach down. Raise both legs at the same time, tightening up the glute area, squeezing your butt as tightly as you can, for thirty reps. Feel free to use ankle weights for added resistance.
- **Step-ups:** Using a step bench, step up and down, one leg at a time. Alternate legs, performing twenty step-ups on one leg at a time. Perform three sets on each leg.

**BONUS MATERIAL

How to Set Yourself Up for Success by Mastering Your Mindset

One of the keys to cracking the code and mastering the program is learning how to budget and schedule your time efficiently. Too many times, I have heard the excuse "But I just don't have enough time to exercise or prepare my meals." I am here to say, "Yes, you do, and I will show you how."

First of all, it starts with your mindset. Give yourself an instant attitude adjustment by improving your mindset toward exercising, eating healthy, and making time for yourself. You want to make the shift from "Ugh! I *have* to do this" to "Yay! I *get* to do this!" Change your "I *have* to's" to "I *get* to's," and you will gain a whole new perspective on taking care of yourself.

Look at exercising as a *gift*. You *get* to give fresh blood and oxygen to all of the cells in your body! You will be a healthier and happier person and a better friend to those around you.

Old Attitude & Behaviors	New Attitude & Behaviors
Diet food is expensive, so I will go through the drive-through instead.	Eating out every day ends up costing more than preparing your meals.
It takes too much time to prepare my meals, so I will grab whatever I can find.	I am worth it to allot five minutes to prepare my meals for the day, thus setting myself up for success.
I love socializing with my co-workers at the local restaurant.	I can still enjoy the company of others who share my new, healthy mindset.
The instant comfort that I get from food soothes me.	Emotional eating is something that I have control of. Food does not help solve my problems.
It takes too long to work out—I don't have two hours a day to waste on training.	I have learned you have to train for only forty-five minutes a day, four times a week to achieve your fitness goals, and I am healthier and happier.

**BONUS MATERIAL
How Food Planning Can Help You Save Time

Preparation Is Key

Set yourself up for success by doing small, yet meaningful everyday practices. Creating and enforcing these powerful habits will pave the way to victory!

Food Planning

- Always designate at least one official grocery-shopping day per week. Make sure to go prepared with your grocery list. Try to schedule your grocery shopping at a time when the store is not crowded so you can focus on getting what you need as quickly and efficiently as possible. I like to go early on Sunday morning before church. It's the best time because no one is there, and I get in and out!

- Always designate one or two days a week as your food-preparation days. Measure, cook, and store your food in microwavable or Pyrex containers for the days ahead. Stack neatly in your refrigerator so you can grab and go. Dry foods such as nuts, cereal, and whole-grain crackers can be measured out and stored conveniently in zip-lock bags.

- Always carry a few highly portable snacks such as fruit or a protein bar in your purse/gym bag so you never go hungry.

- Keep a food journal—this will help keep you on track by reminding you of how far you have come.

- Make a weekly food-planning chart for each day of the week. Map out your week and plug in the meals you plan on eating each day. Although you may not follow this plan to a T, you will go into your week with a game plan.

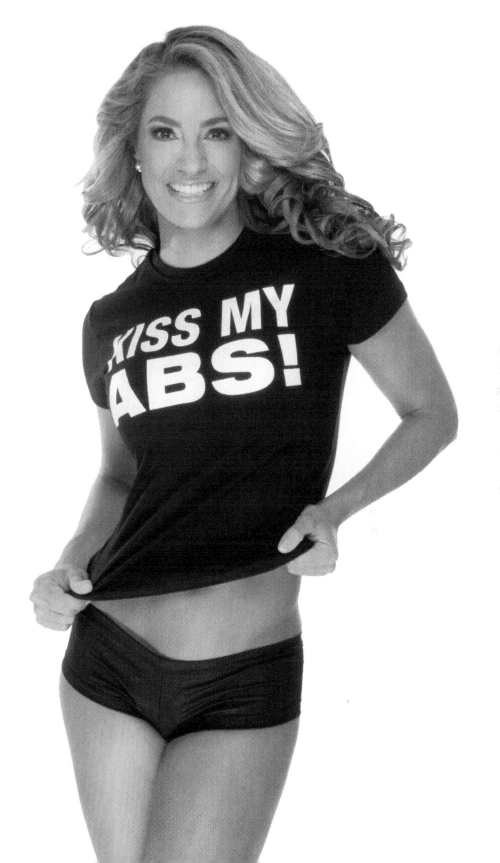

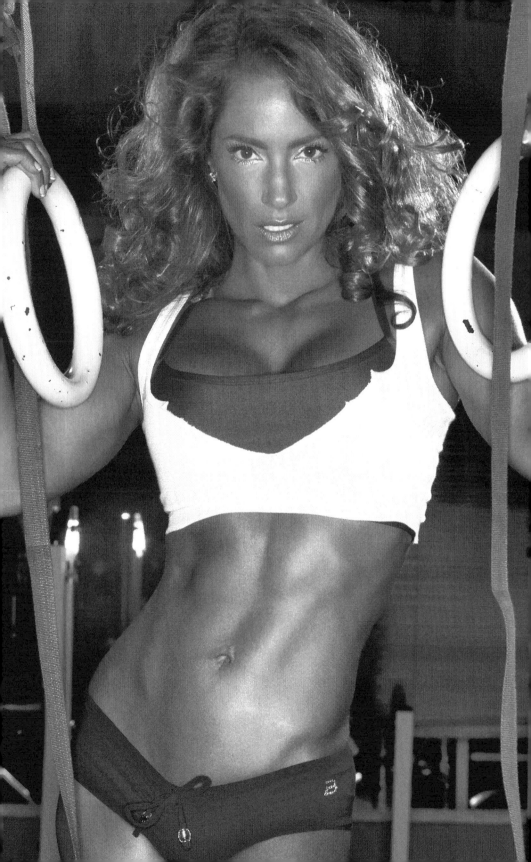

APPENDIX 1

www.fitnessmodelprogram.com

Introducing
The Fitness Model Program™

**This is what you will get with my doctor-approved
Fitness Model Program™:**

• Train like a Fitness Model™
Get max results in minimum time from working out smarter, not
harder!

• Eat like a Fitness Model™
Your body will perform better with more energy, stamina, and
endurance!

• Look like a Fitness Model™
Not only will you turn heads, but you will also break necks!

• Create a beauty regimen like a Fitness Model™
Your hair, skin, and face will represent the ultimate look of health!

• Learn how to banish cellulite forever—it is possible!

APPENDIX 2

www.101thingsnottodo.com

In 101 Things NOT to Do If You Want to Lose Weight™

☑ I **bust** myths of media-promoted fitness crazes such as the low-fat diet.

☑ I **uncover** truths that mainstream media have brainwashed you into believing over the years.

☑ I **reveal** little-known secrets that will *make* or *break* you in your weight-loss journey.

APPENDIX 3

Hollywood's Best-Kept Anti-Cellulite Secret

No one's talking about it, but everyone's doing it! How to fight cellulite and win the war on those darn fat dimples.

https://www.jennifernicolelee.com/JNLSHOP/10Expand. asp?ProductCode=47

Motivate to Lose Weight

If you're stuck in a rut and need a motivational kick in the butt, just listen to lose those unwanted pounds and gain a fresh attitude toward achieving your fitness goals.

https://www.jennifernicolelee.com/JNLSHOP/10Expand. asp?ProductCode=48

Don't Bake It, Fake It!

Learn how to achieve that sexy, golden-bronze glow without the harmful and aging side effects of the tanning bed or sun.

https://www.jennifernicolelee.com/JNLSHOP/10Expand. asp?ProductCode=49

JNL's Extreme Beauty Cosmetic Procedures

The little-known secrets about injectables and full-body treatments revealed! What you need to know about Restylane, Botox, and more!

https://www.jennifernicolelee.com/JNLSHOP/10Expand. asp?ProductCode=50

Supplements for Weight Loss

The "JNL-approved" best fat burners, protein powders, diuretics, and more.

https://www.jennifernicolelee.com/JNLSHOP/10Expand. asp?ProductCode=51

Coconut Oil

The miracle oil that helps you lose weight faster—what you need to know and why you need to start using it today!

https://www.jennifernicolelee.com/JNLSHOP/10Expand. asp?ProductCode=52

How to Look Great Naked

Secrets you can do today to look better in your birthday suit by tonight!

https://www.jennifernicolelee.com/JNLSHOP/10Expand. asp?ProductCode=53

The Real JNL

Her personal struggles and how she overcame them! Her heartfelt story will inspire you to never give up and to keep your momentum in life.

https://www.jennifernicolelee.com/JNLSHOP/10Expand. asp?ProductCode=54

JNL's Success Principles Revealed

Discover the thirty-one top success rules that you need to know to create and enjoy your dream life.

https://www.jennifernicolelee.com/JNLSHOP/10Expand. asp?ProductCode=55

JNL's Eight F's That Equal an A in Weight Training

Learn the tips and tools that you need to know to build sleek and sexy, mind-blowing muscle.

https://www.jennifernicolelee.com/JNLSHOP/10Expand.asp?ProductCode=56

The 411 on the Underwear Fashion Craze of Shape Wear

Discover this super-hot trend that helps remove inches, nip in your waste, smooth out your panty line, and banish that back bra bulge instantly!

https://www.jennifernicolelee.com/JNLSHOP/10Expand.asp?ProductCode=57

The Secrets of Solving Cellulite

Banish the bumps to reveal smooth, sexy legs, butt, and thighs.

https://www.jennifernicolelee.com/JNLSHOP/10Expand.asp?ProductCode=58

Stretch Marks! JNL's Solution

Why we have them, how to prevent them, and how to get rid of them once they show up!

https://www.jennifernicolelee.com/JNLSHOP/10Expand.asp?ProductCode=59

APPENDIX 4

Seven Slimming Secrets to Jump-Start Your Weight Loss Now!

1. Endermologie

Endermologie is the med-spa procedure that actually breaks down fat cells, allowing fat to be flushed out of your system, thus smoothing out the appearance of cellulite and banishing it for good. It does not hurt. In addition, it's been scientifically proven to be as much as 200 percent more effective than a manual massage for releasing built-up toxins and lactic acid.

What to Do: To get more in-depth information on what causes cellulite, and also specific techniques that you can expect in an endermologie session, listen to my Instant Audio Seminar, "Hollywood's Best-Kept Anti-Cellulite Secret: Everyone's Doing It, and No One's Talking about It," here: https://www.jennifernicolelee.com/JNLSHOP/10Expand.asp?ProductCode=47.

2. Detox

No more bloating foods! Stay away from broccoli and brussels sprouts, and opt for asparagus instead! Also, you want to drink citrus water with lemon or lime.

What to Do: Opt for cleansing foods such as cantaloupe, pineapple, watermelon, and honeydews. Also don't underestimate the power of coffee. It's a natural diuretic. If you are sensitive to caffeine, have it in the morning. If you need a stronger diuretic, take an over-the-counter water-shed pill to help you eradicate excess water weight and "pee off the pounds."

3. Stay Away from Sodium

You might be misguided by the thought of soy sauce being calorie free, thinking it's OK to use as a condiment in your diet; however, soy sauce is one of the highest-sodium-content condiments on the market. This means even a touch can lead to a massive five-pound gain of water weight. In addition, your hands and feet can become extremely swollen, along with visibly noticeable puffiness of the neck, jaw, and under-eye area. It can take a good three to five days for your body to purge the physical effects of what soy sauce can do. Soy also raises your estrogen levels. And don't be fooled by light soy sauce; the sodium content is still high!

Olives are heart-healthy but also among the highest-sodium-content items on the market, thus triggering a thirst for liquids, which only adds more water-weight gain! Pickles are the equivalent in sodium content of a bag of potato chips! A pickle is not a *true* vegetable—it is simply a cucumber that has been soaked in sodium and preservatives! Try to steer clear—olives and pickles just dry you up and dehydrate you! *Yuck!* If you absolutely have to have an olive, rinse off the extra sodium.

If you are trying to lean out in a week, make sure you stay away from peanut butter, nuts, cheese, and diet soda, along with all of the other obvious foods that you would not consume if you are dieting.

What to Do: Opt for salt- and sodium-free seasonings such as Mrs. Dash. Opt for a tablespoon of olive oil to reap the health benefits of olives, plus it's great for your hair, skin, and nails. If you get a craving for pickles, choose cucumbers or other precut vegetables with a low-sodium salad dressing.

4. Don't Eat Carbs after 4 PM

Do not eat carbs after 4 p.m. It amazes me how many times I have heard from women in all of my consultations who were still eating carbs after 4 p.m. and expecting to lose weight. I heard so many times that they were consuming pasta, potatoes, breads, rice, and also rolls at dinner, and they could not understand why their weight was not budging.

What to Do: Aim not to eat complex carbs after your late-afternoon snack. You must have a carb at breakfast and for your midmorning snack, then again at lunch, and then again with your late-afternoon snack. The important rule to remember here is not to eat a carb at dinner because, by doing so, you will be working *with* your metabolism rather than against it. The science is simple. If you do eat a carb at night, you will only be storing it on your body, and then your body will have to work harder in the morning to burn it off. I urge you to learn how to "work smarter, not harder" toward your weight-loss goals. By eating a protein and a fibrous carb at dinner (for example, a grilled chicken breast, a green salad, and a serving of steamed asparagus), you will be setting yourself up for success the next day when you are working out, with fewer carbs to burn off!

5. Exercise in the Morning

Don't get me wrong: Exercising at any time of the day is good! It has its health benefits; however, to get the most results and to lose weight more quickly, you should try to work out in the mornings. Exercising at night can sometimes interfere with your normal sleeping patterns because of the spike of energy you get from exerting energy so late in the day.

What to Do: It has been scientifically proven that first thing in the morning is the optimum time to work out because it jump-starts your metabolism!

6. Jump Rope

It's been proven that just ten minutes of jumping rope is the equivalent of running for one hour! It is also a highly portable exercise, so you can do it anywhere!

What to Do: The following is a suggested routine that will help you get the most from your jump-rope workout and have fun doing it:

- Perform one jump-rope exercise for thirty seconds to a minute.
- Rest for a few seconds or until your body feels reenergized.
- Perform the next jump-rope exercise for thirty seconds to a minute.
- Rest for a few seconds or until your body feels reenergized.
- Perform the next jump-rope exercise, and so on.
- For beginners, follow the above pattern for ten minutes. As you progress, work your way up to twenty to thirty minutes for an intense workout.

7. Tan

Use self-tanners! You can actually "tan off" about five good pounds! All fitness models and those in the fitness industry rely on this trade secret. They know that the body looks leaner and more toned with a darker skin color. In addition, your teeth appear whiter, and your skin appears blemish-free when you are tan. Having a tan smooths out acne discolorations, stretch marks, and the appearance of cellulite.

What to Do: If you have more questions, please feel free to take advantage of my super-informative audio seminar titled "Don't Bake It, Fake It! Learn How to Achieve that Sexy, Golden-Bronze Glow without the Harmful and Aging Side Effects of the Tanning Bed or Sun." It's instantly downloadable, and you can listen to it here:

https://www.jennifernicolelee.com/JNLSHOP/10Expand.asp?ProductCode=49

APPENDIX 5

Thirty-One No-Willpower Ways to Lose Weight

1. Have a tea party. Drinking tea daily will hydrate you, keep you feeling full, and give you cancer-fighting antioxidants.
2. Go 80 percent. Eat until you are 80 percent full. It takes the brain twenty minutes to register that there is no more need for food, so stop at a level three of fullness on a scale of one to five.
3. Replace your half-and-half creamer with skim or 2 percent milk.
4. Eat an apple before dinner. It fills you up with good-for-you fiber and will take the edge off a roaring appetite.
5. Become the king/queen of concoctions. Get creative with your favorite cheat food. Mine is nachos with the works, so I use low-fat corn chips, fat-free sour cream, and low-fat cheese instead of the real stuff. I slash the calories without feeling deprived.
6. Cut out the colas. Instead, sip on a glass of fizzy water garnished with a lime or lemon.
7. Instead of one entrée, order two small appetizers. Opt for a house salad with dressing on the side with a bowl of low-sodium soup.
8. When the munchies attack, grab healthy chips. Many now are trans-fat–free and whole grain and may be available in low-sodium versions.
9. Turn up the tunes. It has been proven that music boosts your mood. Therefore, use it to your advantage. Add your favorite songs to your workouts to make them more effective and longer, thus burning more calories and having fun while you do it.

10. Walk. It's free, it keeps you agile and fit, and you can do it anywhere.

11. Replace the candy bowl with a fruit bowl. Vitamin- and fiber-packed fruits will fill you up without the guilt of empty-calorie candy.

12. Use a substitute. Instead of a whole-fat cheese, use low-fat cheese. Instead of ground beef, use ground turkey. You can do the same with hot dogs by substituting the high-fat ones with low-fat, low-sodium turkey hot dogs.

13. Go European with dessert: Delight in a plate of fresh, seasonal fruits.

14. The more colorful your food, the healthier you are—well, with fruits and vegetables, that is. Aim to eat as many different colors as you can to make it fun and interesting while keeping all the taste without the calories.

15. Eat healthy fats to lose fat. Focus on walnuts, avocados, olive oils, and fish containing omega-3 fats. You will shed those unwanted pounds while feeling full and not deprived.

16. Season your way slim. Instead of using butter, salt, and oil and frying foods to make them taste good, stock up on salt-free seasonings and lemon to make your food taste great without all the unnecessary calories.

17. Go darker—with your salad, that is. Instead of the pale iceberg lettuce that has little nutritional value, switch to dark, colorful greens that are vitamin-rich.

18. Chew your calories; don't drink them! Instead of guzzling 300 to 400 calories in about three gulps (Starbucks, anyone?), enjoy chewing and tasting your calories. By sticking with water and forgoing those expensive, high-calorie drinks, you will lose weight for sure.

19. Start grilling and stop frying. Just switching the way you cook or order food can save you hundreds of calories! Opt for a salad with grilled chicken instead of fried, and watch the pounds melt off!

20. Get jumping. It has been proven that jumping rope is one of the most effective and efficient calorie burners that you can do anywhere! Jump ropes are light to pack and fun to use, and jumping rope gives you results.

21. Stop snacking at night. Aim not to eat after 8 p.m. or two hours before your bedtime. If you do get uncontrollably hungry, have a small serving of a high-fiber cereal with skim milk. This will fill you up without derailing your diet efforts.

22. Go nutty. Enjoy a handful of raw, unsalted almonds or walnuts as a snack (about twelve pieces). Nuts are good for you and will cut your hunger pangs in half.

23. Sleep off the pounds. Feeling tired? Instead of grabbing a sugary snack to get you going, take a quick ten- to twenty-minute power nap. You will feel more energized without loading up on calories.

24. Stop stress-eating. When you are pressured, do you reach for food? Start to retrain yourself to solve your problem without the false security of food.

25. Don't commit diet adultery. Cheating means paying for it tomorrow. Remind yourself that an instant on the lips means months on the hips.

26. Get healthy on the go. Stock up on good-for-you grab-and-go foods like celery sticks, low-fat yogurt, and low-fat fiber muffins.

27. Set yourself up for success: Pack a gym bag in your car for your lunch break or for right after work. You'll have no excuse not to go to the gym.

28. Prepare. Prepare. And prepare some more. Plan your meal plans for the next week, do your grocery shopping once a week, and fill your cart with low-fat dairy products, vegetables, lean meats, and fruit.

29. Pee off the pounds. Drink lots of water each day to flush out your system. The water will also make you feel full.

30. Write it down: Keep a food journal, and you will be amazed at all the hidden calories that you are consuming. You will have no more "forgotten" calories when you start tracking what you eat.

31. Defeat the weekend weight gain. We eat more on the weekends! Fight this bad habit by getting moving on Saturday. On Sunday, plan your healthy meals for the next work week ahead.

ABOUT JENNIFER NICOLE LEE

Jennifer Nicole Lee is the CEO and visionary powerhouse behind JNL Worldwide, Inc. Due to her wildly successful, globally broadcasted and marketed fitness and wellness products, books, digital products, e-commerce, and merchandise, she is internationally recognized in over 110 different countries. In short, "JNL" is an extremely successful global megabrand. Mrs. Lee is a fitness celebrity, a bestselling author, a highly sought-after spokesmodel, and the name/face/body of all of her lifestyle brands, wellness products, exercise equipment, DVDs, home, bath, bedding, spa, electronic downloads, and websites. However, and most importantly, she is a devoted wife and mother, representing the millions of other moms and wives in the world with a brand they can trust.

"It's my goal and passion to increase the quality of your lifestyle." —JNL

Jennifer is one of the world's most accomplished Super Fitness Models, and is an international celebrity due to her high-profile wellness merchandise and key media appearances. Jennifer's career as a top fitness expert and icon began when she lost over eighty pounds after the birth of her children. Her motivational weight-loss success story caught the world's attention after she gained accolades as a professional fitness competitor, holding countless titles and crowns. She gained international notoriety, due to her incredible transformation, and was soon a frequent guest on major national talk shows, such as "The Oprah Winfrey Show," E! Entertainment, "Fox & Friends," "Extra,"

"The Secret Lives of Women," and most recently as the top ultimate "pitchwoman" and presenter on Discovery's "Pitchmen," showcasing her captivating and strong TV sales power. Jennifer's energy, creativity, and entrepreneurial spirit, combined with a burning desire to help others, drove her to create the JNL brand. To date she has appeared on a record-breaking forty-four magazine covers.

Some call JNL the female Donald Trump, due to her uncanny ability to brand, promote, market, and sell with the best. Mrs. Lee's passion for business innovation has allowed her to blend lifestyle products and services into the digital realm. Coined as the "Steve Jobs of the fitness industry" she has harnessed the unlimited marketing and sales potential of the Internet, creating a plethora of e-commerce sites, and .com's that rake in a hefty residual income via the world wide web. She is a bestselling author of three hardcover books on diet, nutrition, and exercise, and a contributor to many magazines and eBooks such as *Oxygen*, *Fitness Rx*, and Bodybuilding.com. She also runs an international consultation firm, having coached thousands of women from around the world, and has hosted weekend fitness retreats, drawing women from all over the globe to simply meet her and hear her speak. Jennifer is also a powerful marketing expert, appearing in numerous globally broadcast infomercials for her signature products, including the Ab Circle Pro, Mini Circle, and Chest Magic, and on top shopping networks, such as QVC and the Home Shopping Network. To date, her company and her corporate alliances have three major future lifestyle products soon to be rolling out, with key television media spots secured for advertising. Jennifer is the driving force behind the unprecedented success and future potential of JNL Worldwide.

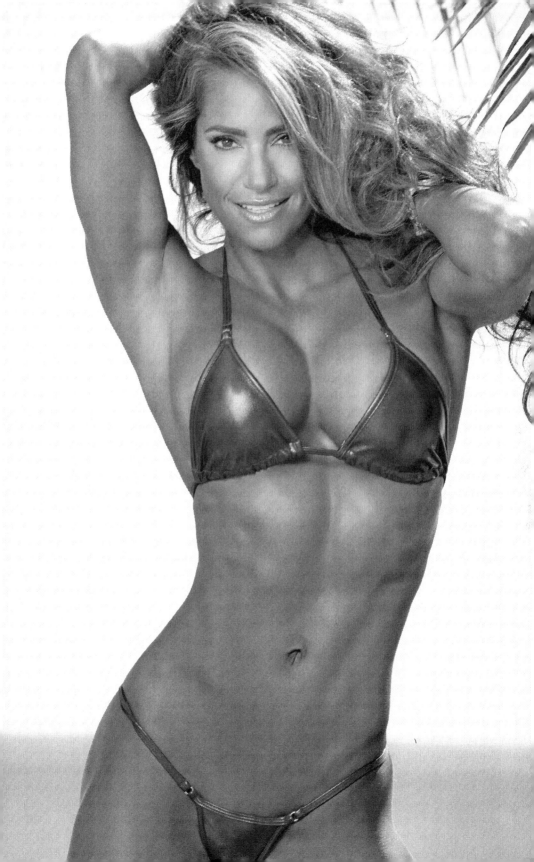

Made in the USA
Charleston, SC
29 December 2014